THE COLON HEALTH HANDBOOK

NEW HEALTH THROUGH COLON REJUVENATION

ELEVENTH REVISED EDITION

Robert Gray

EMERALD PUBLISHING
Box 11830
Reno, Nevada 89510

Author:
Robert Gray
10569 Grand Lake Station
Oakland, California 94610
U.S.A.

Date of first publication, September 1980.

First printing of the Second Revised Edition, May 1981.

First printing of the Third Revised Edition, October 1981.

First printing of the Fourth Revised Edition, April 1982.

First printing of the Fifth Revised Edition, September 1982.

First printing of the Sixth Revised Edition, December 1982.

First printing of the Seventh Revised Edition, March 1983.

First printing of the Eighth Revised Edition, May 1983.

First printing of the Ninth Revised Edition, March 1984.

First printing of the Tenth Revised Edition, April 1985.

First printing of the Eleventh Revised Edition, June 1986.

Printed in the United States of America.

ISBN 0-9615757-1-9

Contents

This book is a synthesis of information gathered from many sources, including modern medical science, ancient Chinese medicine, the Western disciplines of iridology and naturopathy, and the author's personal study, observation, and experience. There are differing views among these various disciplines, and the selection of material in this book does not necessarily fall entirely within the scope of any of them. The conclusions expressed herein are those of the author.

This book is intended for educational purposes, and it should not be used as a guide for the diagnosis and/or treatment of any disease. The reader needing guidance on any particular health-care problem should seek the help of a licensed health-care professional of his or her choice.

Chapter One

Constipation

Nearly every man, woman, and child living in modern society today is constipated. Yes, constipated whether they know it or not. Yes, constipated even though the bowels may move regularly every day. Yes, even people with chronic diarrhea suffer from one form of constipation.

To understand such a statement, consider the meaning of the word "constipate." Its Latin root is "constipare," which means to press together. So constipation is a condition in which one's feces are packed together.

There are two types of constipation. One type is present when the feces that pass from the body are overly packed together. Another type of constipation is present when old, hardened feces stick to the walls of the colon and do not pass out with the regular bowel movements. Both types of constipation are so common among the members of modern society today that scarcely anybody recognizes them as being unnatural. As we shall see, constipated bowel movements are generally looked upon as normal stools. And few people have any inkling as to how much old, hardened feces are chronically present within their bodies.

HOW CONSTIPATION DEVELOPS

Let us consider the operation of the colon. The residues of digested food empty from the small intestines into the colon in liquid form. Muscular contractions along the tube of the colon move the contents of the colon towards the rectum. As this motion occurs, the walls of the colon are constantly at work both absorbing moisture out of the contents of the colon and absorbing waste material from the body into the colon. The longer material remains in the colon, the more moisture is absorbed from it, and the more dry and pressed together it becomes. During a bowel movement, large, powerful contractions called *mass movements* force the contents of the rectum and lower colon through the anus.

The liquid matter out of which the feces are formed may be either thin and watery in consistency or slimy in consistency. A slimy medium will be propelled by the muscular contractions in the colon at a slower rate than will a watery medium. A slimy medium therefore has a longer transit time through the colon. Because it remains in the colon longer, it will have more moisture absorbed from it and be more packed together.

As moisture is absorbed from a slimy medium in the colon, the medium becomes sticky. As the medium is further dehydrated, it becomes gluey and glues a coating of itself to the walls of the colon as it passes through. As layer after layer of gluey feces piles up in the colon, they often form into a tough, rubbery black substance.

Old feces may build up in pockets and they may coat the entire length of the colon and small intestines as well. They do not pass from the body with ordinary bowel movements but require special techniques to dissolve the glue which binds them in the body.

MUCOID VERSUS NONMUCOID STOOLS

The slimy nature of matter found in the colon is due to the presence of mucoid material in what would otherwise be a watery medium. The author terms a stool formed out of mucoid material a *mucoid stool.* A stool formed without the presence of mucoid material the author terms a *nonmucoid stool.*

Because nonmucoid material moves through the body quicker than mucoid material, the bowels tend to move two to three times per day when the intestines and colon are in a nonmucoid condition. The total quantity of feces per day is much greater than when mucoid stools are present because the feces contain much more moisture and are correspondingly less packed together. Because the feces are nonsticky, a nonmucoid stool passes out of the body very easily. The entire contents of a nonmucoid bowel movement usually seems to just drop out of the body within seconds after one sits on the toilet. A healthy nonmucoid stool is neither runny nor mushy. The feces are fully formed as they pass from the body, but, due to lack of any stickiness to hold them together, they may begin to crumble as they rest in undisturbed water. A nonmucoid stool will always break up into little pieces with a small amount of agitation, as when the toilet is flushed.

Because of the longer transit time of mucoid material through the body, bowel movements usually occur no more than once per day when mucoid stools are present. A mucoid stool usually has the appearance of being formed out of lumps that have been pressed together. The more mucoid the stool the more sticky it will be, therefore requiring longer time and more straining to be passed from the body. A mucoid stool will at best only break into chunks when the toilet is flushed.

A *borderline mucoid stool* contains only a small amount of mucoid matter. The bowels will usually move once or twice per day when borderline mucoid stools are present. Borderline mucoid stools never have the appearance of being formed out of segments or lumps pressed together. A borderline mucoid stool requires little or no straining to be passed from the body. It will break up partially but not completely when the toilet is flushed.

In order to judge the mucoid content of a bowel movement, the stools need to be well formed as they pass from the body. Mushy stools will always break up when the toilet is flushed, even though mucoid matter may be present, because they are not dehydrated enough for any possible mucoid matter to become sticky.

Now we can understand why nearly every member of modern society is constipated. The average person has never had a nonmucoid stool since he or she can remember and would think it strange if he or she did. Bowel function is widely considered satisfactory if there is one bowel movement per day that passes from the body within ten minutes. Anytime it takes ten minutes to complete a bowel movement, you are constipated! The feces are probably of a sticky, mucoid nature and have left one more layer of residue inside the colon as they passed through. A bowel movement that takes several minutes to complete may also be due to the presence of much old fecal matter in the colon. This fecal matter can inhibit proper colon functioning and impede the through passage of the fresh feces.

LAXATIVES NOT THE ANSWER

Laxatives merely stimulate the bowels to move. Most operate by irritating the colon, causing the bowels to move until the laxative, together with anything else free enough to flow out, is expelled. There is, however, no specific attempt to expel anything other than the laxative itself. A laxative does nothing to render the stagnant material within the colon free enough to flow out. For this reason, laxatives are of no colon-cleansing benefit.

Once a laxative has passed through the colon, the bowels will still be just as sluggish as ever. Nothing will have been done to remove the accumulation of old feces within the colon. It is this accumulation of stagnant material coating the walls of the colon that counteracts effective colon functioning, thereby leading to a desire to take laxatives. If using laxatives has any enduring effects, they are to weaken the colon from irritation and overstimulation and to cause the body to develop a dependency upon their use.

In order to correct the stagnant constipation chronically present in nearly every person's colon, something much different from a laxative is needed.

What is required is to soften and loosen the old feces present so that they may finally flow out. Doing so is called colon cleansing and is the key, not only to colon health, but to far-reaching health benefits to the entire body as well.

CHRONIC DIARRHEA

There are people with chronic diarrhea who say they are not constipated because their bowels move several times per day. Yes, their daily bowel movements are not constipated, but let us look at the cause of the their diarrhea. Chronic diarrhea is most often due to the presence of irritation in the colon. As long as the irritating influence is present, the colon attempts to expel it by repeatedly emptying itself of whatever can be forced out. In chronic diarrhea, the accumulation of stagnant mucoid, sometimes laden with harmful bacteria or even parasites, is generally of such a magnitude and nature as to be actively irritating. In this case, the source of irritation adheres to the walls of the colon and cannot be expelled. The result is chronic diarrhea. Chronic diarrhea will often respond remarkably to an effective colon-cleansing program.

PARASITES

The discussion of diarrhea brings up the question of parasites because chronic diarrhea is often due to the presence of parasites in the system. Intestinal parasites thrive in filthy environments. The many varieties of intestinal worms lodge themselves in the old matter that encrusts the walls of the intestinal tract. Without the presence of stagnant material to embed themselves in, most intestinal parasites cannot maintain a foothold in the body. Remove this old, putrid, decaying mucoid matter and you will flush the parasites out as well.

MUCOID MANAGEMENT

In the succeeding pages, we show you how to control the mucoid-inducing influences to which your body is subjected and how to use herbal and other countermucoid techniques to lessen their impact upon your body. Once you learn this, you will be able to verify directly for yourself the truth of what is being said. You will find that the greater the balance of countermucoid versus mucoid-inducing influences one day, then the less mucoid will be your stools during some part of the next three days. That is, there will be a tendency towards more bowel movements, faster evacuation, less straining during bowel movements, a less packed together appearance of the stools, and a greater tendency of the feces to break into flakes when the toilet is flushed. Conversely, the greater the balance of mucoid-inducing versus countermucoid influences one day, then the more mucoid will be your stools during some part of the next three days. In this case, there will be a tendency towards fewer bowel movements, slower evacuation, more straining during bowel movements, a more packed together appearance of the stools, and a lesser tendency of the feces to break into flakes when the toilet is flushed.

As we shall see, there are many mucoid-inducing influences to which you and virtually every other member of modern society have been subjected all of your lives. Your colon is, therefore, packed with a lifetime's accumulation of old, hardened feces. As the next chapter shows, this accumulation of stagnant feces within your body acts against good health in several very significant ways. You will never attain superb health before all of the old, hardened feces within your body have been dissolved and removed. In order to become healthy, you must complete the removal of old mucoid matter from your colon.

Chapter Two

The Benefits of Gastrointestinal and Lymphatic Cleansing

In Chapter One, we saw how mucoid material tends to accumulate in the colon. This mucoid material is present throughout the *alimentary* or *gastrointestinal tract*, which extends from the esophagus or food pipe to the anus. Although the colon is the principal location where old mucoid matter accumulates, the walls of the stomach and small intestines do accumulate old mucoid matter as well. *Gastrointestinal cleansing* cleanses not only the colon but the entire alimentary tract.

We have seen how both chronic constipation and chronic diarrhea can arise from a toxic colon, and how colon cleansing can be helpful when such is the case. Let us now explore some of the many other ways the body may be benefited by gastrointestinal cleansing.

MECHANICAL ABNORMALITIES OF THE COLON AND RELATED BODY STRUCTURES

The accumulation of old feces in the colon can and does stretch it and sometimes related body structures out of shape in a number of ways. The colon is made of a series of sacculations or pouch-like segments. At birth these sacculations are all relatively uniform in cross section and are smoothly laid out first as the ascending colon, which extends up the right side of the abdomen to a point near the liver; next as the transverse colon, which extends across the abdomen to a point alongside the left rear of the stomach near the spleen; then as the descending colon, which extends down the left side of the abdomen; next as the sigmoid flexure, which turns toward the center of the body; and finally as the rectum, which connects to the anus. X-ray studies clearly show that, as the colon fills up with old feces, it becomes badly deformed with respect to both its original shape and positioning. Because accumulations of old feces in the colon are virtually universal among the population, mechanical abnormalities are virtually universal also.

When the colon is ballooned, so much old feces may be present that a sacculation has three to four times its proper cross-sectional diameter with only a small channel through which material may pass.

A badly ballooned colon may create so much pressure within the abdomen that part of the gastrointestinal tract protrudes through its normal location within the abdominal wall. Such a protrusion is called a *hernia*. In a *hiatal hernia*, the stomach protrudes up through the opening in the diaphragm where the esophagus or food tube passes. In an *inguinal hernia*, the bulging intestines can be seen as a lump in the groin. Either of these hernias can cause considerable pain and discomfort. In these cases, removing the abdominal pressure by cleansing the colon is an essential step at making it possible for the body to heal itself.

In a *collapsed colon*, one or more sacculations closes in upon itself due to lack of muscle tone in the colon wall. In a *spastic colon*, one or more sacculations is in a constant state of contraction. Where the colon is either collapsed or spastic, it may have one third or less of its proper cross-sectional diameter.

In a *prolapsed colon*, the transverse colon droops or sags. Many times the prolapsus will be advanced enough to put pressure on the bladder, uterus, or prostate, causing trouble in one or more of these organs also.

A *redundant colon* has become so elongated that a section folds back upon itself. This usually severely restricts the passage of feces through, thereby intensifying the rate at which old feces are accumulating.

In *diverticulitis*, the colon wall develops a small outpouching or *diverticulum* that becomes inflamed. In *diverticulosis*, many diverticula are present in the colon.

Hemorrhoids are swellings formed by varicose veins at the anus. They are usually easily aggravated by even small amounts of straining during a bowel movement. In order to permanently overcome hemorrhoids, it is first necessary to progress to the point where one consistently passes nonmucoid stools that flow easily from the body without straining. Secondly, a proper diet must be eaten so as to correct the stagnant toxicity present in the varicose veins.

All mechanical abnormalities of the colon and related body structures—ballooned colon, hernia, collapsed colon, spastic colon, prolapsed colon, redundant colon, diverticulitis, diverticulosis, and hemorrhoids—begin with a toxic condition present in the colon. Colon cleansing is the first and most important step when using natural methods to help the body overcome these problems.

Even after the colon is cleansed, a proper diet and many years are necessary for the colon to regain its proper shape, positioning, and tone. In many cases, colon cleansing alone may be sufficient to end any disturbing symptoms due to mechanical abnormalities.

NUTRIENT ABSORPTION

The accumulation of mucoid material along the walls of the small intestines can interfere with nutrient absorption even though nutritional intake may be adequate. The nutrients that suffer the most are the large molecules, namely, the proteins, vitamins, and enzymes. When such is the case, a person may experience some improvements in physical well-being by supplementing his or her diet with concentrated proteins, vitamins, and enzymes. The improvement is usually relatively short-lived because, except for yeast and spirulina plankton, all of the protein supplements on the market today are highly mucoidforming. The increased mucoid soon thickens the accumulation of material lining the alimentary tract. This further decreases nutrient absorption, so that the individual now needs to further increase supplement intake just to keep his or her state of well-being at status quo. And as protein intake is continually increased, it burdens the digestion more and more, so that a weakened digestion eventually results.

This negative spiral can be escaped by applying the proper solution to the problem. Remove the accumulation of material lining the alimentary tract, and the body will be able to function as designed, utilizing the nutrients available from whole foods alone.

Improving nutrient absorption is much more effective than taking all the known nutrients in supplement form. There are only sixty or so nutrients known to be essential to human nutrition. It has been shown that a diet consisting solely of generous quantities of every known nutrient cannot maintain health. This is because whole foods contain many valuable nutrients not yet isolated or discovered by laboratory science. By taking supplements, we can only get the advantage of a fraction of what the body needs to maintain health. Cleansing the gastrointestinal tract so as to improve nutrient absorption, however, makes it possible to get the full advantage of the complete spectrum of nutrients provided by Nature in whole foods. It is common for a person who has performed the gastrointestinal cleansing program outlined in this book to notice that he or she is then able to eat lighter, more easily digestible foods and smaller quantities of food while feeling more completely satisfied than before.

AUTOINTOXICATION

Autointoxication is the process whereby the body literally poisons itself by maintaining a cesspool of decaying matter in its colon. This inner cesspool can contain as high a concentration of harmful bacteria as a cesspool under a house. The toxins released by the decay process get into the bloodstream and travel to all parts of the body. Every cell in the body gets affected, and many forms of sickness can result. Because it weakens the entire system, autointoxication can be a causative factor for nearly any disease.

Putrefaction

The cause of autointoxication is putrefaction within the intestinal tract. *Putrefaction* is a process of decay in which foul odors and toxic substances are generated. Ideally, there should be little or no putrefaction happening within the body. That is, daily bowel movements should have very little or no putrefactive odor, and there should be no stagnant putrefactive material within the alimentary tract.

The amount of putrefaction present in the body depends upon how long the food undergoing putrefaction has been in the body, upon the efficiency of the digestive processes, and upon what kind of food is undergoing putrefaction. The length of time food stays in the body depends upon two factors—stagnation and transit time.

Stagnation

Stagnation is the failure of matter in the alimentary tract to continue moving until expelled through the anus. When material becomes lodged in the alimentary tract, it can continue to putrefy and release toxins for weeks. Stagnation occurs primarily in the colon and is usually the body's largest contributor to putrefaction and the consequent autointoxication. The primary objective of colon cleansing is to remove stagnant material from the colon and entire alimentary tract. Doing so will sizeably reduce putrefaction and autointoxication within the system.

The stagnant material in the alimentary tract can be divided into two types—putrefactive and postputrefactive. *Putrefactive* matter is still moist, decaying, and releasing toxic substances. Unless removed it eventually becomes so dry and hard that it does not putrefy any further. This *postputrefactive* matter is very difficult to dissolve or remove.

Parasites

It has already been mentioned that worms live in and thrive upon stagnant putrefactive matter within the intestines. Rid yourself of this noxious material, and you will rid yourself of these parasites as well.

Transit Time

Transit time is how long it takes after food is eaten until its residues are expelled through the anus. The shorter the transit time, the less the food will putrefy before being expelled from the body, and the less will be the resultant autointoxication. The average transit time for people in our Western civilization is 65 to 100 hours. It takes about 8 hours for food to travel through the stomach and small intestines, and the remainder of the transit time is spent in the colon. At the end of the colon-cleansing process, transit time may improve to as little as 24 to 48 hours provided a proper diet is eaten and a healthy concentration of lactobacteria is maintained in the colon. The improvement in transit time reduces putrefaction and the resultant autointoxication, and it suggests improved digestion and nutrient absorption, whereby the body processes its food in a shorter amount of time.

How Foods Eaten Affect Putrefaction

The tendency of a food to putrefy or spoil in the body is parallel to that of the same food outside the body. If you let fresh fruit sit outside the refrigerator, it usually takes several days before it begins to spoil. At the same temperature, fresh vegetables will usually spoil in less time than fresh fruit. Unrefrigerated milk usually spoils faster than unrefrigerated vegetables. Unrefrigerated raw meat will spoil in less than a day's time. Moreover, cooking any food generally causes it to spoil quicker than it would if left raw. Because the temperature inside the alimentary tract is in the vicinity of 100° Farenheit, putrefaction of food within the body takes place much more rapidly than at normal room temperature.

In Chapter One, we saw how a mucoid condition within the colon slows the transit time of matter through that organ. The same is true of a mucoid condition within the rest of the alimentary tract. A slimy condition within the small intestines slows digestion and nutrient absorption, thereby increasing transit time. Those foods that putrefy quickly, such as meat, fish, eggs, and pasteurized dairy products, are also high in mucoidforming activity. It is desirable for these foods to pass through the body quickly because of their high rate of putrefaction, but instead they pass through relatively slowly due to their mucoidforming activity. Vegetables and fruits, on the other hand, putrefy relatively slowly and pass through the body quickly due to their easy digestibility and freedom from mucoidforming activity. As a result, the putrefactive impact upon the body of meat, fish, eggs, and dairy products is manyfold that of fruits and vegetables.

It is possible for food to pass completely through the body without putrefying whatsoever. Some time ago, the author read a book that told of a yogi in India who passed perfume-scented feces from his body. At the time, I thought this phenomenon was due to special spiritual powers or was at least a sign of high spiritual development. I later duplicated the result in my own body while eating a diet of 100% raw fruit. After a few days on this diet, my stools lost their putrefactive odor and began to smell like whatever fruit I had eaten several hours before. During this time, my perspiration also had a fruity, somewhat perfume-like scent. The lack of putrefactive odor in my feces was due to the fact that it takes longer for raw fruit to putrefy at 100° Farenheit than the time spent in transit through my body. Also of importance is that my body had been cleansed of stagnant putrefactive material prior to performing the fruitarian diet.

Colon Cleansing Always Necessary

There are many vegetarians who feel that, because so many years have elapsed since they ate meat, their colons must be relatively free of putrefactive wastes. These people should understand that any food, including fruit, will putrefy if held in the body long enough. What causes food residues to be held in the body is the presence of mucoid matter. As mucoid matter is dehydrated in the colon, it turns into a sticky, gluelike substance that tends to hold the residues of all food eaten within the body. You can eat all the fruits and vegetables you want, but if you also eat even relatively small quantities of dairy products, tofu, white flour products, and other mucoidforming foods, the accumulation of putrefactive wastes in the colon will continue.

Those rare people who do eat a totally nonmucoidforming diet also need to remove the accumulation of waste that took place before their diet improved. A nonmucoidforming diet will gradually remove stagnant putrefactive matter from the colon. The most hardened and intractible substances present in the colon, however, are the postputrefactive feces, which have finished putrefying as much as they ever will. These cannot be removed by diet alone. Even after many years on a nonmucoidforming diet, one will still be holding large amounts of old, hardened postputrefactive feces in the colon.

The author is not advocating that everyone eat a totally nonmucoidforming diet. It is commendable if you do, but most people do not. It is advisable, however, that you periodically cleanse your colon so as to keep the accumulation of toxic material at a low level.

Body Odor Can Indicate A Toxic Colon

There is a close relationship between body odor and putrefaction within the intestinal tract. Overall body perspiration, with the possible exception of underarm perspiration, should not create a body odor problem for the person who bathes regularly. The person who cannot control overall body odor no matter how frequently he or she bathes invariably has a highly putrefactive colon. The person who develops overall body odor after a single day at normal room temperature without vigorous activity may also harbor considerable putrefaction within the colon. This does not mean that people who do not perspire readily necessarily have low levels of putrefaction in their colons. These may simply be cases in which the odor does not get out because the perspiration is blocked.

A good indicator of intestinal putrefaction is foot odor. After a typical person wears closed shoes with socks for just one day's time, the socks will be quite smelly. Were the same person to cleanse his or her colon and eat a diet low in putrefactive activity, he or she would find the same socks would accumulate less odor after being worn consecutively for three days than they originally did in one day.

The last body odor to go is underarm odor. Even after the colon is cleansed, most people will still need to use an underarm deodorant. If underarm odor can ever be overcome without the use of antiperspirants or deodorants, doing so requires not only is colon cleansing, but also a long history of body purification dieting and adherence to a totally putrefactive-less food intake.

About The Intestinal Bacteria

The bacteria present in the intestinal tract are generally of two different types. First there are the putrefactive bacteria. The most common species of putrefactive bacteria is *Escherichia coli.* When viewed under a microscope, many putrefactive intestinal bacteria have a characteristic shape or form like that of Escherichia coli and so are called *coliform bacteria.* It is interesting to note that Escherichia coli and other coliform bacteria produce a substance known as ethionine, which has been shown to cause cancer in laboratory animals. Putrefactive bacteria produce a number of other toxic substances as well, including *indole* and *skatole.* These foul-smelling substances give feces their characteristic odor, and their derivative, indican, may be found in the sweat and urine.

Counterbalancing the putrefactive bacteria in the intestinal tract are what has been referred to as the "friendly bacteria." These produce primarily lactic acid, but also acetic acid, digestive enzymes, and vitamins as well. The lactic-acid-producing members of the health-enhancing intestinal bacteria or "friendly bacteria" are know as *lactobacteria*, and include various species belonging to larger groupings named *Lactobacillus, Bifidobacterium,* and *Streptococcus.* The two best know and perhaps most important species of lactobacteria are *Lactobacillus acidophilus* and *Bifidobacterium bifidus.* The name lactobacteria derives from the combining form "lacto-," meaning milk, because these bacteria were first known as the agent responsible for the souring of unpasteurized cows' milk. The so-called lactobacteria are abundantly present on every blade of grass, as well as on mostly all vegetables and grains. That cows eat grass accounts for the presence of lactobacteria in their milk.

The digestive enzymes produced by the friendly intestinal bacteria both aid the digestive efforts of the body and act to control the activity of the putrefactive bacteria. When the putrefactive bacteria become highly active, they emit foul-odored gases in addition to the nongaseous toxins they constantly produce. These gases are usually expelled through the anus, whereupon they are called *flatulence* and create much social embarrassment. If the alimentary tract is so sluggish or obstructed that the gas is not expelled quickly, some of it can become absorbed into the bloodstream, causing headaches and other ill feelings. Both the digestive enzymes from the friendly bacteria and the digestive juices of the body act to inhibit the production of gas by the putrefactive bacteria. Neither will, however, kill putrefactive bacteria or keep them from producing poisonous nongaseous substances.

According to Dr. John Harvey Kellogg, this country's foremost pioneer of colon health, the bacteria in a healthy colon ideally should be 85% lactobacteria and no more than 15% coliform bacteria. Yet we find that the typical colon bacterial count in our society shows only 15% lactobacteria and a monstrous 85% coliform and other types of putrefactive bacteria. This is just the reverse of what it ought to be. No wonder the misery caused by autointoxication is so great and problems with flatulence are so frequent!

A common procedure when flatulence is a problem is to constantly ingest large quantities of lactobacteria-containing foods such as yogurt, kefir, acidophilus milk, acidophilus culture, etc. (The word "acidophilus" refers to *Lactobacillus acidophilus*, which is the best known of the various species of lactobacteria.) Flatulence arises when one or more of the digestive organs— stomach, small intestines, pancreas, liver, or gall bladder—is undersecreting digestive juices, or a duct carrying digestive juices from the liver, gall bladder, or pancreas is partially or completely blocked. Even when the alimentary tract is highly laden with putrefactive bacteria, a well-functioning digestive system will still be able to prevent malodorous flatulence. The practice of blaming flatulence on a "lactobacteria deficiency" seems justified because maintaining a high lactobacteria intake will provide symptomatic relief. Granting that lactobacteria deficiencies are common, we see that they cannot be permanently corrected by ingesting large quantities of lactobacteria-containing foods because the symptom (flatulence) reoccurs within a few hours after the intake of lactobacteria stops. If, however, one cleanses his or her gastrointestinal tract of stagnant putrefactive material, the body, with the help of a proper diet, will then be able to maintain close to the ideal ratio of 85% lactobacteria to 15% putrefactive bacteria without the continual ingestion of lactobacteria-containing foods. In addition, gastrointestinal cleansing is an important first step in correcting the functioning of the digestive organs.

A less-known but equally important function of the friendly bacteria within the intestinal tract is to provide important nutrients for building the blood. Many cases of "tired blood" would benefit more by taking steps to insure a continual high concentration of beneficial bacteria within the intestinal tract than by taking iron tonics. A healthy intestinal flora will produce several times as much of many B vitamins as are present in a well-balanced whole-food diet. This includes vitamin B-12, which is essential for preventing and overcoming pernicious anemia. Some nutritionists argue that an adequate supply of vitamin B-12 cannot be obtained without eating meat. Such a viewpoint does not take into account that cooking meat destroys up to 85% of its vitamin B-12. Since no one eats raw meat, meat cannot be a reliable source for this vitamin. The most abundant source of vitamin B-12 is a healthy intestinal flora. As mentioned above, a toxic intestinal tract cannot maintain a high concentration of live lactic-acid and vitamin producing bacteria, even when lactobacteria-containing foods are being eaten. Once the intestinal tract has been cleansed, however, it is then possible, with the help of a proper diet, to maintain several times the former concentration of lactobacteria without the continual ingestion of lactobacteria-containing foods.

The author is not in favor of the unrestricted long-term use of acidophilus culture, yogurt, kefir, and other fermented foods unless prepared daily at home. They are far too high in lactic acid. Many books and articles will tell you that it is the lactic acid secreted by the lactobacteria that suppresses the gas-producing activity of the putrefactive bacteria, but this is not so. As already noted, the flatulence-suppressing aspect of the lactobacteria is their production of digestive enzymes and not of lactic acid. You do not need lactobacteria to produce lactic acid. Lactic acid is a common end-product of human metabolism that your body cells produce. Scientists have known for a long time that lactic acid tends to build up in the muscles of the body, causing stiffness and pain. And cattle have been known to die of lactic acid poisoning when fed a diet low in roughage and too high in concentrated carbohydrates. The fatal lactic acid was produced by the large amounts of lactobacteria present in the animals' stomachs. In human beings, however, the vast majority of lactobacteria present reside in the colon, where the lactic acid produced is mostly not absorbed into the bloodstream, but serves to hold extra moisture in the feces, making them bulkier and easier to expel. But when lactic acid is ingested through the mouth, it will be absorbed into the bloodstream where it can cause trouble if the quantity is large enough.

When a substance is freshly fermented with lactobacteria, the amount of lactic acid present is relatively moderate and the level of live lactobacteria is high. As time progresses, the level of lactic acid rises rapidly and that of live lactobacteria decreases sharply until, in just a few days' time, there are little or no live lactobacteria left. Even under refrigeration, the ferment will continue to mature, although at a slower rate than at room temperature. When the concentration of lactic acid becomes high enough, the lactobacteria die of autointoxication because lactic acid is excrement and, as such, is poisonous in high concentrations. When supplementing one's diet with lactobacteria, the ferment should be prepared daily at home, then refrigerated, and consumed within 24 hours. Doing so will maximize the live lactobacteria and minimize the lactic acid consumed.

In Chapter Six, we shall discuss how to prepare and use lactobacteria ferments.

LYMPH DETOXIFICATION

When waste material leaves the body cells, it is carried away by the two circulating body fluids, namely, the blood and the lymph.

The lymph is formed out of the blood but contains no red blood cells. Each cell in the body is bathed by the *interstitial fluid,* which consistes of materials from the bloodstream together with substances passed out of the cells. About 90% of the water and small molecules entering the interstitial fluid from the bloodstream are reabsorbed by local blood vessels. The remaining 10% of the water and small molecules plus the protein, other large molecules, and particles in the interstitial fluid collect in a network of tiny lymph vessels. The lymph vessels combine into larger and larger ducts that eventually empty back into the bloodstream. The lymph vessels contain one way valves and are lined with muscle tissue that pumps the lymph through these valves. Because the lymphatic system carries away toxins from all body cells, its proper functioning is important to the health of the entire body.

It is the author's belief that the colon is the principal organ through which mucoid matter from the lymph is eliminated, even though this idea would be quite new in orthodox medical circles. The idea came to me from the recently deceased Loren Berry, who was perhaps the greatest of all manipulative healers of our time. He taught a technique called lymph drain massage, which he credits to have originated from ancient Chinese medicine. Lymph drain massage is to be performed whenever there is an acute sickness, such as a cold, fever, flu, et cetera. Not long after receiving a lymph drain massage, a person will often have a bowel movement in which large quantities of pale-colored mucoid substance is passed. Furthermore, when the sinuses or chest areas of the respiratory system are congested, this effect is more likely to be produced together with substantial relief from the congestion; it is as if a stopper were pulled and the mucus congestion in the respiratory system actually drains out through the colon. Later I discovered that skin brushing, which is explained in detail later in this book, produces the same benefits and effects as lymph drain massage. It also came to my attention that there is a Western science of lymph drain massage poineered by a Dr. Emil Vodder of Denmark.

The science of anatomy reveals that the walls of the colon contain microscopic lymph vessels which combine into larger vessels that empty into the *cisterna chyli*, which is a central lymphatic pool located in the abdomen. Lymph from the small intestines, back, and lower body also empties into the cisterna chyli. The cisterna chyli is the origin of the *thoracic duct*, which travels up the body and connects with the bloodstream slightly below and to the left of the base of the neck. Through the thoracic duct, lymph from all parts of the body, except the right side of the head, neck, and chest and upper right arm, empty into the bloodstream. Most physiology textbooks state that the lymph flows only in one direction—away from the colon and other tissues, into the cisterna chyli, and from there back into the bloodstream through the thoracic duct. How then can we account for the large amounts of pale mucoid substance subject to be present in the colon after lymph drain massage or skin brushing?

In my research to answer this question, I discovered three scientific facts. First, a Dr. Olszewski of Poland has observed with the use of scientific instruments that the kind of stimulation to body surfaces provided by skin brushing does in fact stimulate the flow of lymph. Second, the lymph can and does undergo *retrograde flow*, which is a flow in the direction opposite to that which is considered normal. Third, a particular type of retrograde flow called *chylous reflux* has been observed wherein lymph flows from the cisterna chyli back into the colon or other body tissues. Chylous reflux to date has only been medically observed when the body is under the stress of disease. This is not surprising, however, because medical science concerns itself only with disease states.

Physiology texts usually discuss no purpose for the cisterna chyli, but the author submits that it may serve to collect mucoid material carried away from the body cells by the lymph and direct it into the colon, so that only the watery portion of the lymph is passed into the bloodstream. Otherwise, the blood might become too thick to circulate.

The remainder of this section on Lymph Detoxification is based on the author's extensive personal observations and experience, which totally supports the conclusion that the colon serves to detoxify the lymph. I find that an unobstructed colon will absorb the mucoid material in the lymph through its walls into its interior. As the walls of the colon become more obstructed with linings of fecal deposits, however, its ability to detoxify the lymph decreases and the accumulation of mucoid matter begins to back up into the lymphatic system, and congestion of the lymphatic system can result.

A toxic lymph is usually present during an acute sickness. It sets the stage for disease by hampering the activity of the white blood cells, which must fend off invasions by pathogenic elements. White blood cells are found in the lymph and interstitial fluid and can move about under their own power of locomotion. Without being carried by the circulation, they can move in a straight line from one body part to another by squeezing in between the body cells. When the lymph is toxic, both it and the interstitial fluid become thick and viscous. Thinning the lymph and interstitial fluid by using lymph-purifying herbs can greatly improve the mobility and disease-fighting effectiveness of the white blood cells. Many herbal procedures for acute sicknesses are centered around either bayberry bark or lobelia, both of which are lymph purifiers.

Very often in acute sicknesses, the appetite is lost and the body metabolism goes into the fasting mode. In the fasting mode, all body cells throw off toxins at an increased rate. Many of these toxins are forced into the lymph, where a mucoid substance is formed to hold them in suspension. When the lymphatic system becomes extremely full of mucoid material, a pressure is created that is felt all over the body. It starts as a tension in the muscles that becomes an aching of the muscles as the pressure increases. One function of a fever is to thin the lymph mucoid, thereby improving its ability to flow and to pass through the walls of the colon. All lymph-purifying influences reduce fever by lessening the necessity for using fever to thin the lymph.

If the colon cannot perform the necessary rate of purification of the lymph, then the body uses the liver to do the work instead. The toxins taken up by the liver are excreted as part of the bile. When the flow of bile becomes excessive, bile backs up into the stomach, and the result is nausea.

In Chapter Six, we will give an acute-sickness procedure based upon the remarks in this subsection. It is interesting to note that most grasses are lymph purifiers, and this explains why animals eat grass when sick.

In the preceding section we discussed autointoxication, which is due to the accumulation of putrefactive matter in the intestinal tract. In this section, we are concerning ourselves with the results of the accumulation of postputrefactive matter in the colon. It is mainly this postputrefactive matter that compromises the ability of the colon to detoxify the lymph.

Now we can see how problems can originate when the colon becomes clogged. When this happens, waste material gets backed up into the lymphatic system. As this process continues, waste material backs up into the body tissues and disease can result. This process can affect any body part because the lymphatic system serves all body cells.

Cleansing The Lymphatic System

The first step in cleansing the lymphatic system is to cleanse the colon so that the excess mucoid material backed up in the lymphatic system can be drained out.

The second step in cleansing the lymphatic system is to practice skin brushing. This is a highly effective technique for stimulating the expulsion of fresh mucoid material, hardened particulate or impacted mucoid matter, and other obstructions of the lymphatic system and for correcting inflammations of the lymph nodes. Like the colon, the lymphatic system can contain stagnant accumulations of old waste matter. Once the colon is at least partially cleansed, it takes a few months of daily skin brushing to completely cleanse the lymphatic system. Detailed instructions for performing skin brushing will be given in Chapter Five.

When practiced daily for several months, skin brushing is very effective for improving body tone. Five minutes per day of skin brushing is easily worth thirty minutes of vigorous physical exercise in this respect.

Lymph mucoid will often begin to appear in one's stools as soon as colon cleansing proceeds far enough to relieve the pressure from the mucoid matter backed up in the lymphatic system. To completely cleanse the lymphatic system of all stagnant material, however, skin brushing must be continued for some period of time.

When present in sufficient quantity, lymph mucoid can be easily seen in one's stools. Its general appearance is like that of petroleum jelly, although it may vary in color from practically clear to dark brown. Lymph mucoid may have a jellylike consistency rather than the sticky consistency of the alimentary tract mucoid. It may pass through the colon with little tendency to cause constipation and be expelled before it becomes appreciably dehydrated. When lymph mucoid does get trapped in the colon, it eventually hardens along with the rest of the stagnant material.

Once the lymphatic system has been purged of stagnant waste material, its healthful functioning can be assured by keeping the lymph pure on a day-to-day basis. This can be done by keeping the colon clear and nonconstipated, regular skin brushing, and avoiding the excessive intake of mucoidforming foods. Even once cleansed of stagnant material, the lymphatic system can become overladen with fresh lymph mucoid in a day's time, just as a cleansed colon can become constipated again in a day's time. Proper health care is a day-to-day affair.

REFLEX MAPPING

Not too many years ago, few people in this country had heard of acupuncture or acupressure. Today, state legislatures are moving to license the practice of acupuncture as a bona fide healing art. The basic idea is simple. Stimulating a specific body point by sticking a needle into it or even by applying mechanical pressure to it will favorably affect the health of a remotely located body organ or part. Conversely, when a body organ is in distress, the acupuncture point or points related to that organ will be tender or painful to the touch.

Some body parts are unique in that they contain a reflexly related point for every other body part. The feet and the hands both have this property. We express these relationships by saying the feet map the entire body and the hands map the entire body.

Also mapping the entire body is the intestinal tract. Every point along the intestinal tract is reflexly related to a specific body part. A toxic condition at one point of the intestinal tract can and does produce ill health in its reflexly related body part. When disease in a body part stems from a toxic condition of the associated reflex center in the intestines, then the single most important factor in overcoming that disease is to detoxify the intestinal reflex center. In practice, the colon is usually much more toxic than the small intestines. Hence, the majority of diseases arising from a toxic condition in the intestinal tract have their source in the colon.

Iridological Evidence

The knowledge of how the intestinal tract maps the body has been gained from the science of iridology. *Iridology* is the science and practice of studying the *iris*, or colored portion of the eye, to detect inflammations throughout the body. The iris is a map of the body, and a skilled iridologist can discover many details about tissue conditions all over the body by analyzing the iris.

Figure 1 shows how the right and left irises map the body. Different portions of each iris have been labeled according to the body part to which each corresponds. Encircling the pupil are the small and large intestines. Around these are positioned various body parts. A toxic condition at a given spot in the intestinal tract can cause disease in that body part located radially outward on the chart. For some examples, let us look at the chart of the left iris. The point at which the transverse colon turns and becomes the descending colon is called the *splenic flexure*. From the chart, we see that a toxic condition of the splenic flexure can result in disease in the medulla or mastoid areas. A toxic condition halfway along the descending colon can result in disease of the heart, the lungs, or the bronchials. The point marked "N" refers to the navel. A toxic condition in the navel area can result in disease in the lower back.

Every practicing iridologist repeatedly witnesses the reflex relationships between the intestinal tract and the rest of the body. Many times a person with a disease will report having had pain in the associated intestinal reflex center for years before the disease developed. For example, an elderly woman with cancer of the right breast may report having had pain in the reflexly related portion of the ascending colon most of her adult life.

The Enema Effect

The reflex relationship of the intestinal tract to the rest of the body explains why enemas are often of favorable impact in a wide variety of diseases. The *enema effect* is the reflex activity upon various body parts caused by fluid entered into the body through the anus. Stimulating the colon by means of an enema causes healing reflexes in many parts of the body. Even when little or nothing is rinsed out of the colon, an enema or quick succession of enemas can constitute a powerful impetus for the body

Be Notified
of Additional Activities
# of Robert Gray

Now you can follow all aspects of Robert Gray's work—simply and easily

Each day Robert Gray receives letters from readers of *The Colon Health Handbook*. These people are enthusiastic about his work and repeatedly ask about the availability of additional ways to benefit by his ability to help people. Many sense Robert Gray's commitment to promote better health through wholistic and natural means and would like to see more people touched by his work. Because he knows that there are thousands more people like these, Robert Gray now offers to send to all who are interested in any aspect of his work:

- *Advance notice when new books being written by Robert Gray are completed*

- *Articles and personal messages from Robert Gray*

- *Notification of public and media appearances by Robert Gray*

- *Information on new self-help programs developed by Robert Gray*

- *Information about seminars and trainings when offered by Robert Gray*

- *Ways those interested can participate in Robert Gray's efforts to bring better health to the world*

Identify yourself as a friend of Robert Gray and his work. Your name and address will be kept confidential and will not be added to any other mailing list. Simply fill out and send in this handy card today.

Please Print Clearly

Name _____

Address _____

_____

_____ Zip _____

Fold and then tear along this line

Emerald Publishing

P. O. Box 11830

Reno, Nevada 89510

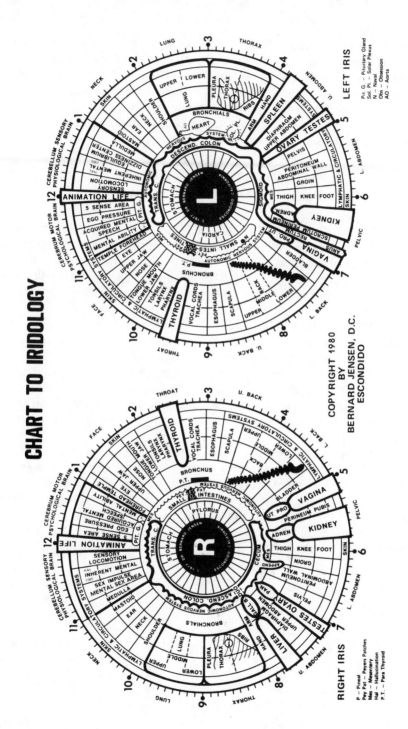

Figure 1. Courtesy Dr. Bernard Jensen. Reprinted by permission.

to heal itself.

Many of the beneficial effects of colonic irrigations are due to the enema effect. Colonic irrigations are actually enemas given with continuously running water which enters the body at the same time waste is being expelled. It is widely believed that the effectiveness of colonic irrigations lies solely in their ability to remove stagnant putrefactive matter from the body. However, a colonic irrigation that removes little from the body can still have a powerful impact.

GASTROINTESTINAL CLEANSING AS PREVENTIVE HEALTH CARE

This chapter shows that the overall health of the body is intimately connected to the condition of the gastrointestinal tract in general and of the colon in particular. Indeed, there are many authorities who claim that virtually every disease begins with a toxic colon. While the truth of such a statement is difficult to judge accurately, it can be said with certainty that a toxic gastrointestinal tract can be a factor in the causation of nearly any disease. While gastrointestinal cleansing alone is not a cure for any disease, the body will be able to overcome any disease more easily once the gastrointestinal tract and lymphatic system have been cleansed.

You have no way of knowing exactly how much of the physical suffering you have been through so far could have been averted had you kept your alimentary tract cleansed. You can be certain, however, that the longer you let its unhealthy condition go uncorrected, the more you are eventually going to suffer for it.

In the past, colon cleansing was difficult, time consuming, and/or expensive. Now this book can help you attain the far-reaching preventive health-care benefits of gastrointestinal and lymphatic cleansing with little inconvenience and at a moderate cost. The program outlined herein is more comprehensive and effective than any other method. Many people have found it has helped them to feel twice as good in just sixty days. But in order to benefit from it you must act. You must carry through with the full course of this gastrointestinal and lymphatic cleansing program.

Chapter Three

The Mucoid Question

In Chapter One, we saw that the accumulation of old feces in the colon was due to a mucoid condition in the alimentary tract. In this chapter, we will give the information promised in Chapter One which will allow a person to test for himself the connection between mucoidforming influences and constipation.

THE MUCUS CONTROVERSY

Most everybody has experienced that, if one spends enough time in a dusty air environment, one will eventually cough up some thick mucus with dust particles trapped in it. The mucus is used as a method of entrapping a potentially harmful substance so as to prevent it from penetrating deeper into the body, and as a medium for expelling this substance from the body.

From the above observation, it would seem plausible that, if the body responds to the ingestion of a particular food with the production of mucus, then that food contains some substance the body recognizes as potentially harmful or toxic. In this line of thought, any food that has "mucusforming" properties is considered to be potentially toxic to some degree.

The *mucus theory*, which holds that mucusforming foods are potentially toxic, has long been a hotly debated issue. As we shall now see, the source of the controversy is mainly poor communication and poor understanding about the processes involved.

As far as the author is concerned, the validity of any theory should be judged by its usefulness in predicting what will actually happen in practice. In Chapter Two, we discussed in detail the harmful effects of constipated feces remaining stagnant in the colon. Any food that has a tendency to produce constipation or stagnation must, therefore, necessarily be considered potentially toxic.

Sources Of Poor Understanding About The Mucus Theory

In attempting to test the validity of the mucus theory, most people look for mucus in the respiratory system and not in the stools. Testing for mucusforming activity through the respiratory system is highly unreliable because the respiratory system will produce mucus with some mucusforming foods and not others and at some times and not others. People never think to look for evidence of mucus in their stools because, in most cases, they do not even know what it is not to have mucus present there. The person who wants to test the validity of the mucus theory must first improve the balance of countermucoid versus mucoidforming influences until he or she finds out what a nonmucoid stool is. At this point, one can then test for the mucusforming activity of what are known to be mucusforming foods.

Mucus is a normal body secretion. All mucous membranes continually secrete mucus as a means of keeping the surfaces moist and lubricated. Ingesting any food, or even water, will give rise to an increased level at the back of the mouth of a healthy, lubricating type of mucus. These facts are often presented as disproving the validity of the mucus theory. Yet it is easy to distinguish healthy mucus from mucus formed as a reaction to toxicity. Healthy mucus is clear and slippery. Unhealthy mucus is cloudy, thick, and sticky, and this is the type of mucus produced by mucusforming foods. The difficulty encountered here between proponents and detractors of the mucus theory lies in the area of communication and terminology. Some proponents of the mucus theory prefer to use the word "catarrhalforming" instead of "mucusforming" because "catarrh" refers to an inflammation of a mucous membrane, and so clearly points to an unhealthy condition. Perhaps there is wisdom in this because all foods, and even water, produce mucus of the healthy type. Most proponents of the mucus theory consider the healthy type of mucus to be not mucus at all, but merely a normal body fluid. On the one hand, detractors of the mucus theory have defined mucus as any secretion of the mucous membrane, while, on the other hand, the proponents have implicitly defined mucus as a morbid secretion of the mucous membrane. At any rate, the important thing to know is that the healthy type of mucus does not call attention to itself. There is probably some mucus of the healthy type in what the author has termed a nonmucoid stool, but it is completely nonsticky and unobtrusive. Whenever there is noticeable mucus in the respiratory system, or whenever discernably mucoid stools are present, you can be sure that a potentially toxic condition is being indicated.

Oftentimes proponents of the mucus theory will refer to the body tissues as being saturated with mucus, to mucus being present in the lymph, etc. These expressions are well understood by almost any person who speaks English as his or her native tongue. Yet according to modern scientific definition, mucus is a secretion of the mucous membrane. Because there is no mucous membrane tissue in most body muscles or in the lymphatic system, there could not be any mucus there. Many a usage of the word "mucus" that is correct in common parlance will be contradictory or incorrect according to the meaning of the word as a precise scientific term.

Even so, we must remember that the word "mucus" was part of the English language with its existing common usage long before modern scientific conventions were set. "Mucus" originated as a Latin word which was later absorbed into the English language.

There is a disease which medical science calls "myxedema." In this disease, the body swells up with a solution of what biochemists identify to be *mucopolysaccharides*. The word "myxedema" is derived from the Greek roots "myxa," meaning mucus, and "oidema," meaning a swelling. So, literally, "myxedema" means a swelling with mucus. But to say that in myxedema the body swells up with mucus is scientifically incorrect because mucopolysaccharides are not mucus.

The author does not question the need for precise definitions in an exacting field such as biochemistry. There are myriads of substances present in the body. In order to unravel the complex functioning and interaction of these substances, it is essential to be precise when using terminology. My only regret is that the word "mucus" came to be defined in a way that is so often at odds with its traditional usage.

In a book such as this, the author is not trying to communicate with biochemists and other life scientists. The aim here is to communicate to the common person what he or she needs to know about proper health care. To use precise technical terminology in such a discussion would only overwhelm the average person and defeat the purpose of what is being said.

Mucoid Matter Defined

In order to avoid the many semantical difficulties associated with the word "mucus," the author prefers to use the expression "mucoid matter" instead. "Mucoid matter," "mucoid material," and "mucoid" all refer to any slimy, sticky, or gluelike substance originating in the body for the purpose of holding substances to be eliminated in suspension. The term generally encompasses what the ordinary English-speaking person would accept as being mucus whether the actual substance be mucus, mucin, colloid, mucopolysaccharides, mucoproteins, glycoproteins, or what have you. Mucoid matter may be formed in the respiratory system, alimentary tract, lymphatic system, uterus, vagina, urinary system, connective tissue, or other body part and may be present in or exude from any body tissue. Slippery but nonsticky substances found within the body for the purpose of providing lubrication, such as the normal mucus that forms at the back of the mouth when one drinks water, are by definition not considered mucoid matter. Also excluded from the definition of mucoid matter are mucopolysaccharides and other constituents of mucoid matter when present in forms not possessing the consistency and function of mucoid material.

MUCOIDFORMING INFLUENCES

About Dietary Change

Although excessive comsumption of mucoidforming foods and inadequate levels of intestinal lactobacteria are the principal causes of a toxic colon, the author does not recommend that you immediately switch to a totally nonmucoidforming diet. Both the body and the psyche need time to adjust to any dietary change. Remember, a pendulum that swings far in one direction will eventually swing far in the opposite direction. If you rush into abruptly eliminating foods from your diet, then you will eventually feel so uncomfortable that you will begin eating those same foods again. In changing your diet, the object is to avoid the pendulum effect. Be gentle with yourself. Never try to eat in a way that feels forced. Make a firm resolution to improve your diet, and then keep your goal in thought while you patiently look for ways to comfortably satisfy that goal.

In general, the author recommends that you proceed at whatever pace feels comfortable to gradually eliminate most mucoidforming foods from your diet while replacing them with nonmucoidforming ones. This evolution may take place over the course of several weeks or of several years. How far you want to go is up to you. Some people will eventually make all of the recommended changes, some people half, some a fourth, and some none of the changes. However, performing the author's gastrointestinal cleansing program provides an ideal opportunity for you to make dietary change because doing so will enable you to feel more satisfied while eating much lighter foods than before. Most people feel they could never be satisfied eating just vegetables, fruits, and sprouts, and this is quite true when the intestines are laden with mucoid material. Remove the mucoid from your intestinal tract, and you will be amazed at how substantial and satisfying a diet of primarily vegetables, fruits, and sprouts can be.

The fewer mucoidforming foods you eat, the better the health you will eventually be able to attain. Those who do not want to change their diet at all can still get some benefit by following the author's gastrointestinal and lymphatic cleansing program. Remember, however, that superb health can never be attained as long as a highly mucoidforming diet is being eaten.

Mucoidforming Foods

The rating of foods according to mucoidforming activity is not something you have to accept on blind faith. You can judge for yourself the mucoidforming activity of foods eaten simply by inspecting your stools.

Instructions for doing so have been given in Chapter One.

We are not here going to present a detailed argument in favor of vegetarian eating. Other publications by the author will address the question of proper eating at length, but to do so here would be too much of a divergence from the subject matter of this book. The author is not in favor of eating any animal products, whether flesh foods—meat, fish, and eggs— or dairy products. And I have helped many people a great deal by showing them how to properly avoid these foods. However you react to my position need not stop you from proceeding with my gastrointestinal and lymphatic cleansing program. The purpose of this brief section on foods is not to answer every question you might have about dietary change, but simply to give you enough information to test for yourself the relationship between mucoid stools and mucoidforming foods.

Dairy products from cows' milk, whether pasteurized or raw, are the most mucoidforming of all foods. This includes milk, skim milk, butter, cheese, cottage cheese, cream, yogurt, kefir, ghee, and whey. Every one of these is a pernicious mucoidformer. Goats' milk, however, is substantially less mucoidforming than cows' milk.

Flesh foods—meat, fish, foul, and eggs—are almost as mucoidforming as cows' milk dairy products. They usually affect the respiratory system less but the total amount of mucoid is still quite high.

Plant foods vary from highly mucoidforming to totally nonmucoidforming. Before classifying them according to mucoidforming activity, let us define our terms.

Here we will classify the edible portions of plants as either vegetables, fruits, mature seeds, or sprouts. *Vegetables* are edible roots, trunks, stems, stalks, leaves, flowerbuds, flowers, succulent immature seeds, and single-celled organisms. When a seed is enclosed in a tender, juicy, edible medium, that medium is termed *fruit*. Seeds normally eaten along with the fruit they are imbedded in are considered part of that fruit. *Mature seeds* are divided into oily seeds, grains, and pulses. *Oily seeds* include all nuts and other nutlike seeds such as sunflower, sesame, and pumpkin seeds. *Grains* are the mature dry seeds of plants belonging to the natural order of grasses. Examples are wheat, rice, rye, corn, barley, oats, triticale, and millet. For nutritional purposes, we also classify buckwheat as a grain, although the plant does not belong to the grass family. *Pulses* are the mature dry seeds of pod-bearing plants. These include all beans, lentils, mature dry peas, etc. A *sprout* is the initial developing stage of a new plant obtained when a seed begins to grow. A sprout becomes a vegetable when it is no longer customary to eat the entire plant as a single unit.

Check your understanding of the above definitions with these examples. Pineapple, maple syrup, yeast, and spirulina plankton are classified as vegetables. String beans, cucumbers, okra, eggplant, zucchini, all melons, and all squashes are fruit. Fresh corn on the cob is a vegetable, but corn meal, corn bread, corn chips, and corn tortillas are all grain products. Fresh peas in their tender, juicy state are a vegetable, but mature dry peas, such as are used in making split pea soup, are a pulse. Wheatgrass is a vegetable.

Soy beans are the most mucoidforming of all plant foods. Their mucoidforming activity is similar to that of meat, fish, and eggs and comes close to that of dairy products. The susceptibility of soy products to putrefaction is also similar to that of meat. Notice how quickly tofu or soy milk will spoil. Soy beans have gained much attention as being a nutritionally suitable plant food substitute for dairy products and flesh foods. They are a suitable substitute not only with respect to protein and other nutrient content, but with respect to mucoidforming activity and putrefactive susceptibility as well. The idea that soy beans are favorable to overall nutrition is based upon their similarity in biochemical composition to animal products (dairy products and flesh foods). If you want to improve health by giving up animal products, then you must also give up the nutritional—or rather anti-nutritional—intake associated with an animal product diet. Vegetarians who regularly include soy products in their diets are paying pricely homage to the utterly false and highly injurious idea that their bodies cannot do without animal products.

After soy beans in mucoidforming activity are all other pulses. There is a substantial gap in mucoidforming activity between soy beans and the other pulses. Even so, the mucoidforming activity of the other pulses is considerable. Buckwheat is similar to the pulses in mucoidforming activity.

After pulses in mucoidforming activity are the grains. Next after these are the oily seeds. Millet is a special grain in that its mucoidforming activity is only about one fourth to one third that of the other grains, and so is similar to the oily seeds in mucoidforming activity. Because whole grains are often eaten to assure bowel regularity, it is possible to get the impression that grains are nonmucoidforming, although this is not the case. We shall have more to say about grains and bowel regularity later in this chapter when we discuss bran.

Sprouts lose their mucoidforming activity as the sprouting process continues. When used as a grain substitute, sprouted grains have usually been sprouted for 1½ to 2 days and still have some, though substantially less, of the original mucoidforming activity. To be completely free of mucoidforming activity, the grains, buckwheat, and soy beans typically need to be sprouted for six or more days at room temperature. This is usually done by growing the sprouts in a tray of soil. The young plants are harvested by cutting them away from their roots, so that what is eaten would be classified as a vegetable. Pulses other than soy beans will usually lose all of their mucoidforming activity after three to four days of sprouting at room temperature.

Honey will vary in mucoidforming activity depending upon the plant it is derived from. Most honeys have little or no mucoidforming activity.

Eucalyptus honey is one that is to be noted for its relatively high mucoidforming activity.

Vegetables and fruits are virtually free of any mucoidforming activity. They are Nature's purest foods. Exceptions are gas-ripened bananas and sulphured fruit, which are mucoidforming due to the man-made processes to which they have been subjected. Almost all bananas sold in this country, including most sold in health food stores, have been gassed to induce ripening. On sporadic occasions, one may be able to find non-gas-ripened bananas at certain health food stores. Except for figs and dates, all dried fruit should be considered to be sulphured unless specifically labeled otherwise.

Food supplements are often mucoidforming. All protein powders, except for 100% pure yeast and spirulina plankton, are highly mucoidforming due to their inclusion of soy, milk, egg, or meat derivatives. Many popular "yeast" powders are highly mucoidforming because they contain up to 50% whey. Tableted vitamins, minerals, digestive enzymes, etc. may also possess a degree of mucoidforming activity.

Herbal foods will often alter the mucoid content of one's stools. There are metabolic activator herbs that will lessen the mucoid present in one's stools. There are also many other herbs that, while not mucoidforming themselves, will cause old mucoid present in the body to be eliminated; this may result in increased mucoid in the stools. The jellylike consistency of psyllium husks makes one's feces cling together even when a totally nonmucoidforming diet is being eaten. Many spices possess varying herbal properties; cinnamon and cumin are especially to be noted for their constipating tendency. And the gelatin capsules that are so widely used for encapsulating powdered herbs possess a residuum of mucoidforming activity. In order to avoid biasing the results when testing the mucoidforming activity of ordinary foods, items such as those mentioned in this paragraph should not be taken.

Airborne Mucoidformers

Airborne pollutants are generally all mucoidforming. A sensitive person on a nearly or completely nonmucoidforming diet can notice a significant mucoid response due to breathing smoggy air. The secondary smoke inhalation that occurs when one is present in a room where another person is smoking tobacco is also mucoidforming. The mucoid response to airborne pollutants is frequently more easily noticeable in the respiratory system than in the stools.

Poor Mucoidforming Resistance

Some people are much less resistant to the effect of mucoidforming influences than the normal person. For these people, even minor exposures to mucoidforming food or air may result in a considerable mucoid response. Try as they may at a nonmucoidforming diet, they seldom manage to get a completely nonmucoid stool. These are the people with a low metabolic rate due to insufficient thyroid activity.

Earlier in this chapter we mentioned the existence of the disease myxedema, in which the body tissues become swollen with a mucoid substance. This disease is due to a degenerative condition of the thyroid which results in a very low thyroid output. Without a sufficient thyroid output, the metabolism slows down. Food is incompletely burned, and the result is like smoke or soot as compared to a clean-burning flame. This internal smoke or soot is handled in the same way smoke or soot from the outside is handled. The body generates mucoid material to hold the undesired substances in suspension.

While myxedema is an extreme form of thyroid deficiency having a low incidence among the population, lesser degrees of thyroid underactivity are quite common. In these conditions, the body is less able to metabolize or burn up mucoidforming substances, resulting in more mucoid being produced. The high level of mucoid among the body tissues must drain into the lymph, which easily becomes overloaded when the colon is toxic. Therefore, lymphatic congestion symptoms such as respiratory disorders, urinary system disorders, female disorders, and skin diseases will be present with greater incidence or severity than among those with satisfactory thyroid activity. A low energy level will usually be present and is typically attributed in error to the anemia that is frequently present also. The anemia arises because the ability of the bone marrow to produce blood cells falls rapidly with decreasing temperature. When thyroid activity is low, the body temperature is also low, and the extremities are the coldest. In this situation, there may be little or no blood cell production taking place in the extremities. Other possible symptoms of low thyroid activity are migraine headaches and an increased susceptiblity to atherosclerosis (hardening of the linings of the arteries) with its various resultant forms of heart and circulatory system disorders.

One indicator of metabolic rate is body temperature. Body temperature varies with physical activity but generally increases gradually throughout the course of a day's activities. During sleep, the body temperature falls and usually reaches its lowest point of a 24-hour period just before one awakens at the beginning of the day. The *basal temperature* is the lowest body temperature over a 24-hour time period. It may be used as a test for level of thyroid activity.

To measure your basal temperature, it is best to obtain a basal temperature thermometer. These are commonly sold at pharmacies for use by women in determining their times of ovulation. These thermometers have an expanded scale and possess the high level of accuracy necessary to properly judge the body's metabolic rate. Before going to bed, shake the thermometer down and place it by your bedside. Immediately upon awakening after a night's sleep, place the thermometer under one side of your tongue and lie still with the eyes closed for seven minutes. Then switch the thermometer to the opposite underneath side of your tongue for three more minutes before taking the reading. Do not sit up, get out of bed, toss and turn, drink any fluids, or engage in conversation before taking the temperature, as it will rise quickly once activity of any type begins. Keep taking your basal temperature on consecutive days until you have ten good readings after omitting all readings of whose accuracy you are uncertain. Women should use readings obtained from the start of a period to the day before ovulation, which usually occurs about fourteen days later. At ovulation, the basal temperature drops suddenly to about ½ degree below its average, and then it gradually rises to a peak of about ½ degree above its average one or two days before menstruation.

The normal basal temperature range is 97.8° to 98.2° Farenheit. When the thyroid output is low, the basal temperature tends to flucutate markedly while generally remaining below 97.8°. The metabolic rate changes about ten percent for each degree of temperature. A low basal temperature indicates a slow metabolic rate and a high temperature a fast metabolic rate. Other than during times of illness, nervous tension, or fasting, this test will give an accurate indication of thyroid activity except for about one percent of the cases having a low reading. For these one percent, the low reading will be caused by adrenal deficiency or pituitary deficiency.

COUNTERMUCOID INFLUENCES

Metabolic Activators

Metabolic activators help the body to metabolize or "burn up" mucoidforming substances rather than produce mucoid to hold them in suspension. There are two possible modes for this kind of activity. One is that of a *thyroid activator,* which promotes increased thyroid output, thereby raising the metabolic rate and improving mucoidforming resistance. The second is one that acts directly on the body tissues at the cellular level to promote increased metabolic activity.

It is widely presumed that any substance which raises metabolic activity is therefore a thyroid activator. The author, however, has never been able to verify thyroid-activating properties for any substance tested. If we take a metabolic activator and prepare a lotion from it, we can then apply this locally to any body part. If the lotion contains thyroid-activating properties, we would expect a much larger effect from applying the lotion to the thyroid area of the neck than from applying an equal amount on a distant body part, such as a leg. It must, of course, also be true that the total amount of active ingredient entering the body through an application is less than that required to be in the bloodstream to produce the maximum possible effect. In making the test, the author has never been able to produce the expected results. Instead, I have found that preparations of metabolic activators will often produce a local warming sensation immediately upon application through the skin. This suggests that most metabolic activators are in fact not thyroid activators.

Let us now discuss some metabolic activators. They are mostly useful as an adjunct to an already effective weight-loss program, as they help to burn calories a little more quickly. They are not of value, however, for the long-term control of mucoid within the intestinal tract because the body very quickly develops homeostatic resistance to them in this respect. As discussed in Chapter Five, *homeostatic resistance* is the body's activity of nullifying the effect of a substance to which it is regularly exposed. We discuss metabolic activators mainly for the sake of completeness.

Bladderwrack (Fucus versiculosis (Linn.); Fucaceae): This seaweed is very potent for raising the metabolic rate. Its only common herbal use is for losing weight. In overdoses it is prone to produce tenseness, nervousness, heart palpitations, and emotionality. It is difficult to use, as its dosage must be individually determined for each person. Although the chemical analysis has never been done, the author believes that the chemical structure containing the iodine in this seaweed is closely allied to some part or all of the thyroid hormone. Note: If you have a low basal temperature, do not try to treat yourself with this herb, especially if you have a history of any type of atherosclerotic-related disease. There are intricacies to handling these conditions with thyroid hormone that require the skill of a physician. The author believes that people with low thyroid activity can enjoy good health without the use of thyroid hormone if they respect their situations by eating a diet especially low in mucoidforming activity, keeping the colon and lymphatics clean, and maintaining a healthy population of lactobacteria in the colon.

Oatstraw (Avena sativa; Graminaceae): A very small amount per day is sufficient to produce the maximum possible metabolic activator effect. In larger dosages, it acts as an appetite-suppressant as well as a metabolic activator, making it ideal for losing weight. Its appetite-suppressant activity is much more certain than that of chickweed, which is the most commonly used herb for this purpose. Oatstraw is very powerful for detoxifying the joints in the body, but it acts in such a way that a highly toxic joint may become painful as the toxins are being removed. Its virtues have often gone unappreciated because it needs to be boiled twenty to thirty minutes in order to extract its active principles.

Spirulina plankton (various Spirulina species; Algae): Here is another metabolic activator that is also an appetite suppressant and therefore good for losing weight. It is very energizing, being generally superior to all ginsengs, dong quai, bee pollen, and vitamin B-15 in this respect. The combination of spirulina's energizing and appetite suppressant properties has made it popular for use while fasting. Spirulina is an aggressive cleansing herb that empties toxins out of the body tissues into the lymph. A highly toxic lymph or painful joints may result from using spirulina in too large of a dose or over too long a period of time. Aggressive cleansing herbs are discussed in the next chapter. They are useful for ridding the body of toxic wastes but must be used carefully and properly if side reactions are to be avoided.

Grapes, raisins, and grape juice: All varieties of grapes possess a good amount of metabolic activator activity. Grapes and raisins are aggressive cleansers which, if eaten in too large a quantity, can aggravate a toxic joint.

Irish moss (Chondrus crispus (Stackh.); Algae): This herb is often used for controlling halitosis or bad breath. It will decrease the depositing of the whitish scum or plaque that coats the tongue and teeth. It is often included in herbal preparations intended to act on the thyroid, but the author does not know that it has such an effect.

Yeast (Saccharomyces cerevisiae) and vinegar: These two items are similar in effect. Vinegar must be undistilled to contain the active principle. Apple cider vinegar is the common item specified for health-enhancing purposes, but rice vinegar and wine vinegar are undistilled also. The metabolic activator properties of yeast and vinegar are usually used for weight loss, and both have, perhaps erroneously, been referred to as activators of the thyroid.

About Kelp

This seaweed is widely taken as an aid to the thyroid. It is a good source of iodine, which the thyroid needs for proper functioning, and it also provides other valuable minerals, but has no metabolic activator properties. When a low thyroid output is due to a dietary deficiency of iodine, then kelp, or any edible seaweed for that matter, will solve the problem. But when a low thyroid output is due to a hormone imbalance in the body or to a weakened condition of the thyroid gland, more than kelp alone will be needed to remedy the situation.

The Intestinal Lactobacteria

A healthy population of lactobacteria within the intestinal tract far outstrips all metabolic activators known to the author as far as controlling the mucoid content of one's stools is concerned. In fact, it is generally not possible to obtain a nonmucoid stool without a healthy population of lactobacteria in the intestinal tract. The presence of these lactobacteria promote bulky, well-lubricated stools as well as more frequent bowel movements. Unlike the metabolic activators, lactobacteria are not subject to the body's homeostatic resistance.

The lactobacteria and putrefactive bacteria in the intestinal tract contrast with and counteract each other in various ways. Lactobacteria live on carbohydrates, whereas putrefactive bacteria live on protein. Putrefactive bacteria do not grow well in the acidic medium produced by lactobacteria. However, the metabolization of protein by the putrefactive bacteria produces ammonia, which neutralizes the acidity produced by the lactobacteria. It therefore takes a vigorous growth of lactobacteria in the intestinal tract to finally predominate over the putrefactive bacteria. A high-protein diet will always produce large amounts of putrefactive bacteria in the intestinal tract even when the diet contains substantial amounts of carbohydrates as well.

The bowels will normally be slow to move unless the contents of the colon has reached a certain acidity. The colon is in fact a bacteriological fermentation chamber, and it is as if the body judges when the ferment is mature by the acidity within the colon. When the colon contains large amounts of lactobacteria together with relatively low levels of putrefactive bacteria, the acidity will be such that the bowels move two to four times per day. When such is the case, the feces will have spent a relatively short period of time in the colon, and so will have a high water content, making them soft and bulky when expelled.

Lactobacteria feed off of many different forms of carbohydrates. However, a high-carbohydrate diet alone is not necessarily sufficient to insure a healthy population of lactobacteria in the intestinal tract. This is because the lactobacteria must compete with the body for the carbohydrates eaten. When food is swallowed, it goes first to the stomach where it is held for awhile in a highly acidic medium while protein digestion is begun. The high acidity is not essential to the protein digestion, but does act to destroy most of the bacteria present in the stomach. When food leaves the stomach and enters the small intestines, the live bacteria count is nearly insignificant and the body then reverses most of the acidity towards alkalinity. As the food travels through the small intestines, the bacterial count increases very slowly. Not until the food residue empties from the small intestines into the colon is it ordinarily exposed to large populations of bacteria. If the body absorbs nearly all of the carbohydrates eaten by the time the food residue empties into the colon, a healthy population of lactobacteria cannot be maintained in the system, and the putrefactive bacteria will dominate. This can happen because protein, which feeds the putrefactive bacteria, is much more difficult to digest and assimilate than carbohydrates, and so will always be present in the food residue.

Two foods are deserving of special mention for their ability to greatly assist the lactobacteria at predominating over the putrefactive bacteria in the intestinal tract. The first of these is cabbage. Cabbage selectively feeds lactobacteria; they thrive and grow quickly on it. At the same time, cabbage tends to suppress the growth of putrefactive bacteria. When used daily for several days, and provided sufficient lactobacteria are present in the body, cabbage not only counteracts intestinal mucoid but also sizeably reduces the putrefactive odor of one's bowel movements. To obtain a noticeable effect, it is necessary to drink ½ to 1 cup of cabbage juice two to three times per day. It may be sweetened with maple syrup or honey if desired. Whole cabbage has the same effect as cabbage juice. One pound of cabbage per day must be eaten to have a sizeable effect.

The second food deserving of special mention is the sun choke. Sun chokes are sometimes also referred to as "Jerusalem artichokes." However, the sun choke is a tuber which grows underground and bears no resemblance in appearance to an artichoke. When cooked, however, the taste is somewhat similar. Sun chokes were little known in this country a few years ago, but are becoming increasingly more widely available. They contain a carbohydrate called *inulin*, which is not digested nor absorbed by the human body. There are species of lactobacteria, however, which do feed on inulin. When sun chokes are eaten, the inulin they contain serves as a source of lactobacteria food for which the body does not compete. Most of the inulin eaten reaches the colon intact. An enormous amount of lactobacteria growth can be supported by a relatively small intake of sun chokes.

In common nutritional practice, it is thought that either lactose or dextrin must be ingested when it is desired to provide a lactobacteria food that will not be digested and absorbed by the body. Lactose is a dairy product; it is often eaten in the form of whey, which contains lactose. Dextrin is a man-made carbohydrate. Both are highly mucoidforming. The sun choke, however, is a nonmucoidforming food which serves the same purpose. The author is the first nutritionist to discern the value of the sun choke as an alternative to lactose, whey, and dextrin.

Sun chokes may be eaten raw or cooked. When eaten raw, they may be grated or sliced into wafers and included in a salad. To cook sun chokes, steam them in wafers with other vegetables or bake 1½ hours at 350° F (175° C). Only 3 to 4 ounces (75 to 100 grams) of sun chokes per day are needed to insure an abundant growth of lactobacteria in the intestines, provided, of course, a beginning population of lactobacteria is already present. While sun chokes are a much more potent lactobacteria food than cabbage, they do not possess the power of cabbage for reducing putrefaction in the intestinal tract.

Dietary Fiber

Dietary fiber is the indigestible portion of the food we eat. Much attention has been given lately to the benefits of dietary fiber upon colon functioning. These beneficial effects derive from several different modes of activity, and different forms of dietary fiber possess different combinations of these modes of activity. Some forms of dietary fiber are helpful to colon functioning because they hold extra moisture in the intestinal tract. Some forms of dietary fiber benefit colon functioning by providing a bulky mass which increases the ability of the intestines to move its inner contents along. When consumed in adequate amounts, many forms of dietary fiber aid in supporting a plentiful population of lactobacteria in the intestinal tract. As noted above, a healthy population of lactobacteria is of paramount importance for controlling the mucoid content of one's stools. In order for the countermucoid effect of many forms of dietary fiber to be significant, there must first be a good implantation of lactobacteria in the intestinal tract. The fiber then acts to keep the lactobacteria at a high level of activity and to avoid their extinction.

Another important benefit of many varieties of dietary fiber is that they lower the levels of either or both of two fatty substances in the blood known as *cholesterol* and *triglycerides*. High levels of cholesterol or triglycerides in the blood represent greatly increased risk of heart or circulatory system disorders, and any factor that can significantly reduce the blood levels of either of these is considered to be highly beneficial to good health.

Some of the best forms of dietary fiber are sprouted legumes, cabbage, carrots, and millet. They contain a relatively large amount of fiber that has a high biological activity. Meat, fish, foul, eggs, dairy products, white flour, white sugar and other refined carbohydrates contain virtually no dietary fiber.

About Bran

Bran consists of the tough, indigestible coatings of edible grains. The principal sources of the bran present in the average whole-food diet are whole wheat and whole corn. Rice, rye, oats, and millet have less bran than these two. Barley contains such a thick bran that only pearled barley, which has had some of the bran polished away, is sold for human consumption. Wheat bran is commonly sold as an individual substance. Those who supplement their diet with it do so in order to benefit colon function.

Even though eating bran can produce looser stools, the author is not in favor of it as one's principal source of dietary fiber for several reasons.

One objection of the author to bran stems from the high levels of a substance known as *phytate* present in commercially availabe wheat bran. Phytate has the capacity to bind calcium and magnesium present in one's diet in such a way that these minerals become unavailable for absorption. The phytate present in wholemeal flour has been related to the negative calcium balance that develops in people living largely on wholemeal bread.

Researchers also think that phytate impairs the absorption of iron and zinc. Commercially available wheat bran typically contains over 80% of all the phytate present in the whole grain.

A second reservation the author has with respect to wheat bran is its mucoidforming activity. Although wheat bran can produce a sizeable reduction in mucoid present in the colon, it does so, in the author's observation, at the expense of creating more mucoid in other parts of the body.

A third disadvantage to the use of wheat bran as a source of dietary fiber is that it does not lower blood cholesterol levels, as do many of the vegetable and fruit fibers.

People who habitually rely upon eating bran or large amounts of whole grains in order to avoid feeling constipated would do better to abandon this practice in favor of, first, consuming generous amounts of fiber from vegetables and sprouts and, second, maintaining a healthy population of lactobacteria in the intestinal tract. Any form of bran will produce looser stools and propel them from the body more forcefully. A moderate amount of bran, as may be present in a well-balanced whole-food diet, will usually not be harmful. But when bran in any form becomes necessary to insure normal bowel function, the proper solution to this problem should be implemented.

Negative Ions

Negative ions are molecules that carry an electrically negative charge. They can be present in gaseous, liquid, or solid mediums. As far as aiding health is concerned, the discussion of negative ions refers mainly to those present in the air we breathe.

Ions in the air are created by cosmic rays and radon gas, both of which are everywhere present in the lower atmosphere. These influences cause ordinary air molecules to split into pairs of a negative ion plus a positive ion. Negative and positive ions rarely stay evenly mixed in the atmosphere. Air near the surface of the earth typically contains somewhat more positive than negative ions, while air high above the earth's surface frequently contains more negative than positive ones. Lightning occurs when the charge carried by a concentration of negative ions in a cloud discharges to the ground. At high mountain altitudes, moreover, electrical conditions can sometimes be such that negative ions predominate in the air near the earth's surface. Storms and fast-moving water such as waterfalls and bubbling creeks can also cause negative ions to predominate in the air in their vicinity.

A major significance of negative ions is their ability to remove smog, cigarette smoke, pollen, dust, harmful bacteria, viruses, and other pollutants from the air. When air contains more negative ions than positive ones, tiny airborne particles suspended in it will acquire a negative charge. When this happens, their static electricity causes the particles to coagulate into large enough clusters to fall from the air. The result is air that is more pure than normally encountered.

Breathing this clean air is exhilarating and refreshing. It is the experience of crisp, fresh air that occurs near waterfalls and just after a thunderstorm. Inhaling it while asleep can produce feelings of deeper sleep and of being more refreshed upon awakening.

When positive ions predominate over the negative ones, little cleaning of the air takes place. Air pollution, electronic equipment, air conditioning, air heating, falling barometric pressure, and hot, dry seasonal winds all produce excess positive ions, which deplete the air of its negative ions.

By removing pollutants from the air, we can greatly reduce the amount of toxicity that enters our bodies. Most people do not realize how much toxicity they take in through breathing. When a whole-food diet of low mucoidforming activity is being eaten, smoggy air can easily contribute the major portion of all mucoidforming activity. A few minutes of breathing air cleaned by negative ions can even lessen or end an asthma or hay fever attack.

MUCOID A UNIVERSAL PROBLEM

Mucoid is a universal problem in our society. Virtually everybody has eaten a highly mucoidforming diet since the age of weaning. Furthermore, modern-day air is typically laden with mucoidforming pollutants. As a result, mucoid production in your body has proceeded at a high level throughout your life. Over the years there has been a gradual accumulation of stagnant mucoid within your system, which in various ways has caused you repeated and increasingly severe trouble. Even people convinced that they now eat a healthy diet will continue to harbor large amounts of stagnant mucoid until definitive steps are taken to remove it.

The program given in this book shows the starting point for ridding your body of its accumulation of stagnant mucoid. Although the accumulation has taken place throughout your system, the largest deposits by far are in your colon. Because stagnation in the colon eventually backs up into the lymph and all the body tissues, colon cleansing is the first step at correcting the mucoid condition present in your body. There are few if any diseases against which your body's fight cannot be benefited by gastrointestinal and lymphatic cleansing. Detailed instructions that only take a few minutes per day to carry out are given in this book. An ounce of prevention is worth a pound of cure. Take that small step towards the far-reaching protection of your body against sickness, disease, and suffering. Receive the benefits you seek to obtain in reading this book. Carry through with the gastrointestinal and lymphatic cleansing program outlined herein.

Chapter Four

Mucoactive Herbology

Mucoactive herbology is the science of how herbs may be used to affect mucoid within the body. An *herb* is any plant or plant part capable of having a significant impact upon health when ingested or otherwise applied to the body in an amount too small to be considered significant as food. An *agent* is an herb, food, or other bodily influence that has an impact upon health common to that of a particular category of herbs. For example, an antimucoid agent is any bodily influence whose activity is like that of an antimucoid herb.

From what has already been said in this book, it is obvious that using herbs to cleanse the colon and lymphatics is an exercise in mucoactive herbology. There are many mucoactive herbs, and the subject of mucoactive herbology is too vast to be fully explored here. We will, however, try to present enough of this intriguing subject to create an understanding of herbal gastrointestinal and lymphatic cleansing. Of the number of different possible modes of mucoactivity, we shall here discuss the mucotriptic, deobstruent, lymphatic-cleanser, mucosynergistic, mucoaggressive, muco-corrective, and antimucoid ones.

MUCOTRIPTIC HERBS

Mucotriptic herbs loosen, soften, or dissolve hardened, stagnant, or impacted mucoid in the body. "Mucoid" is a general term encompassing a number of chemically different substances. "Mucotriptic" therefore denotes a broad category because not every mucotriptic herb will attack every variety of mucoid. There are both broadly acting mucotriptic herbs capable of affecting most mucoid found within the body as well as mucotriptic herbs whose activity is specific to certain conditions or body parts. In gastrointestinal cleansing, mucotriptic herbs specific to the gastrointestinal tract are useful for removing large amounts of hardened mucoid from the gastrointestinal tract while avoiding the difficulty arising from simultaneously dissolving considerable amounts of mucoid throughout the body.

While mucoid can accumulate in any body part, the three areas where mucoid tends to accumulate most are the gastrointestinal tract, the lymphatic system, and the joints. All three of these areas are primary sites for mucoid generation. The cartilage present in a joint contains mucous membrane cells for generating a clear and slippery mucus that keeps the joints lubricated. When mucoidforming substances are present, these cells emit a sticky, toxic mucoid that builds up deposits within the joint.

Mucotriptic herbs that act upon the mucoid present in the gastrointestinal tract are called *deobstruents*. Mucotriptic agents that act upon the lymphatic system are called *lymphatic cleansers*. Skin brushing is the most effective lymphatic cleanser known to the author. While there are many lymphatic cleansing herbs, their effectiveness is usually poor compared to that of skin brushing.

Some mucotriptic agents are acacia gum, aloes, balm of gilead buds, barberry bark, bayberry bark, chickweed, chives, corn silk, elecampane root, eyebright, golden seal root, grapes, iceberg lettuce (use or dehydrate before any milky juice or narcotic properties develop), irish moss, jojoba oil, nettles, oatstraw, olive oil, plantain, red clover flowers, rosemary, rue, spaghetti squash, spirulina plankton, tomatoes, violet leaves, white bryony root, yellow dock root, and zucchini. Of these, acacia gum, aloes, barberry bark, bayberry bark, chickweed, chives, corn silk, golden seal root, grapes, iceberg lettuce, irish moss, olive oil, plantain, red clover flowers, rosemary, spirulina plankton, white bryony root, yellow dock root, and zucchini are deobstruents.

SYNERGISM

Synergism is the co-operative action of two or more agents wherein the total effect is greater than the sum of the effects of the agents used separately. *Mucotriptic synergism* or, more simply, *mucosynergism* is a synergism of mucotriptic agents. It is of key importance for herbal gastrointestinal cleansing. The author knows of no single herb that will completely cleanse the gastrointestinal tract when used alone, no matter for how long a period of time. In fact, the deobstruent properties of some herbs listed above as deobstruents cannot be discerned unless the herb is used as part of a mucosynergistic combination.

The fact that mucoid deposits are mixtures of many different substances helps to explain the phenomenon of mucosynergism. Let us suppose a hardened material contains a group of substances called "A" and a group of substances called "B." Then the mixture of a strong solvent for group A but not group B plus a strong solvent for group B but not group A will have more solvent activity on the hardened material than the sum for the solvents used separately.

A *multisynergistic* herb will form synergistic combinations with many different herbs. The most important multisynergistic herb known is lobelia. Lobelia has been recognized as a virtuous herb since 1793, but modern herbology has Dr. John Christopher to thank for his diligent work at making its synergistic importance widely appreciated. And now the author submits that the second most important multisynergistic herb is plantain (Plantago major or P. lanceolate (Linn.); Plantaginaceae). This is actually a multimucosynergistic herb, as it will augment the activity of many different mucotriptic herbs. When plantain is used alone, its mucotriptic activity is significant but not extraordinary. Yet when used mucosynergistically, it can change a good herbal formula into an excellent one.

PURIFYING THE LYMPH

Lymph-purifying herbs lessen the amount of mucoid present in the lymphatic system. This is usually accomplished by thinning the consistency of the lymph mucoid so that it will pass into the colon more easily. Stimulating the muscles that pump the lymph along the lymph vessels will also have a lymph-purifying effect.

Most lymph-purifying herbs have no antimucoid activity. The difference between an antimucoid herb and a lymph-purifying herb is that one acts before and the other after mucoid has been created. An antimucoid herb gets rid of mucoidforming substances before the mucoid is created, while a lymph-purifying herb moves the mucoid out of the lymph once it has been created. A lymph-purifying herb will not make the stools any less mucoid unless it also has antimucoid properties. Many antimucoid herbs are also lymph purifiers.

Purifying the lymph and cleansing the lymphatic system are different processes. "Purify" is being used in the sense of removing impurities, as from a solution. "Cleanse" is being used in the sense of breaking down, dissolving, and flushing away hardened material. To cleanse the lymphatic system means to mobilize and remove hardened, sedimentary, and impacted matter and to relieve all lymph tissues from inflammation. This typically takes several months. To purify the lymph just means to insure the watery rather than mucoid consistency of the lymph fluid. This can often be accomplished in a few hours. The difference between a lymph purifier and a lymphatic cleanser is like that between paint thinner and paint remover. Paint thinner only acts on fresh paint, while paint remover dissolves dry, hardened paint. Because lymphatic cleansing is the more thorough process, lymphatic cleansing influences such as skin brushing will also have a lymph-purifying effect, but lymph purifiers will usually not be lymphatic cleansers.

The purity of the lymph may vary constantly and can change markedly after a meal. Even once the lymphatics have been cleansed, the lymph constantly needs to be kept pure because there will be a constant flow of waste material from the body cells into the lymph. Keeping the colon unobstructed is an important step towards keeping the lymph pure because doing so lessens the resistance to the passage of mucoid out of the lymph.

Most lymph-purifying herbs increase the toxicity of the blood in the course of purifying the lymph. This is because the majority thin the lymph mucoid so that it will pass more readily into the colon. Doing so, however, dissolves some of the toxins being held by the lymph mucoid into the lymph fluid, which empties into and becomes part of the bloodstream. Lymph-purifying herbs having this type of activity are best combined with an appropriate amount of blood-purifying herb so that the blood will be simultaneously purified rather than made more toxic.

Some lymph-purifying herbs are acacia gum, aloes, balm of gilead buds, bayberry bark (powerful), bladderwrack, cabbage, chaparral, chia seeds, couchgrass, iceberg lettuce (powerful—use or dry before any milky juice or narcotic properties develop), irish moss, kudzu, lemon balm, lobelia, oatstraw, oregon grape root, pine oil (small amounts), red clover flowers, sage, sumach bark (powerful), thyme, tormentil root, uva ursi, wheatgrass, white bryony root, wild cherry bark, and yeast. All of these increase the toxicity of the blood except for acacia gum, balm of gilead buds, cabbage, chaparral, couchgrass, iceberg lettuce, lemon balm, oregon grape root, and uva ursi.

THE DYNAMICS OF HERBAL USE

Over the last several decades the practice of medicine has been dominated by allopathic modalities. *Allopathy* is the treatment of disease using remedies whose effects are immediately opposite to the effects of the disease being treated. For example, an allopathic approach may call for giving pain killers when there is pain, giving fever suppressants when there is fever, and surgically removing an organ that is highly debilitated.

Today more and more people are becoming interested in alternatives to allopathic health care. Herbs and other forms of natural healing are receiving growing attention.

While it is possible to use herbs allopathically for symptomatic relief, the majority of herbs operate differently from the majority of pharmaceutical drugs. Most pharmaceutical drugs today have as their principal mode of operation some manner of suppressive activity that counteracts symptom manifestation by lessening a bodily activity. While herbs having suppressive modes of activity do exist, mostly all herbs, on the other hand, possess a mode of activity that in some way moves or affects toxic substances. Nearly every disease has somewhere in its chain of causative factors an interference by toxic substances with proper bodily functioning. When we turn to her for help, Nature, in her wisdom, usually provides something that will act upon the toxic substances that lie at the source of disease. Hence, most herbs possess at least one mode of activity that, in some way, helps to cleanse the body of toxic substances.

Cleansing Reactions

When toxins are moved in the process of cleansing the body, the body may temporarily react to the new distribution of toxic substances within its system with any of a wide variety of symptoms. Such symptoms are known as *cleansing reactions*. An herb that has the potential to produce a cleansing reaction is called an *aggressive cleansing herb*. A few examples of cleansing reactions are skin eruptions, dizziness, disturbed sleep, itching, emotional unrest, and intensification of a preexisting symptom.

While cleansing reactions can take many forms, the mechanisms behind their manifestation are relatively few.

Blood-aggressive herbs increase the toxicity of the blood, and *lymph-aggressive* herbs increase the toxicity of the lymph. As nonmobile toxins are dissolved, they are taken up by the lymph and the blood, which then carry them to the organs of elimination—liver, kidneys, lungs, bowels, and pores—to be removed from the body. If the rate at which toxins are being emptied into the blood or lymph exceeds the rate at which the organs of elimination are removing them, cleansing reactions will result.

Another type of cleansing reaction is a *mucoaggressive response*. An herb having the potential to initiate a mucoaggressive response is called a *mucoaggressive* herb. Mucoaggressive herbs are mostly mucotriptic agents that soften hardened or impacted mucoid without removing it from its location in the body. In the process of being softened, the hardened mucoid swells up with water. This creates a pressure among the tissues which is felt as an active disturbance. Mucoaggressive responses are experienced as pain, stiffness, or swelling in a joint or muscle or as a stabbing sensation among the body tissues. Of the mucotriptic herbs listed earlier in this chapter, most have a mucoaggressive potential. The only ones known to the author to be free of mucoaggressive activity are corn silk, iceberg lettuce, plantain, white bryony root, and yellow dock root.

The cleansing reaction associated with deobstruent herbs is constipated and infrequent bowel movements. As hardened mucoid within the alimentary tract is dissolved, it reabsorbs water and becomes sticky again. When this sticky mucoid mixes in with the material moving through the intestines, there will be a tendency towards longer transit times, which, as explained in Chapter One, will result in more constipated and infrequent bowel movements.

Another cleansing reaction is flatulence or gas. As explained in Chapter Two, the digestive juices of the body act to inhibit the formation of gas in the intestinal tract. The secretions of the liver, the digestive juices from the gall bladder, and the digestive juices from the pancreas all enter the small intestines at a single point through what is known as the common bile duct.

When, in the course of purifying the body, the liver throws off thick, sludgy mucoid matter, this can clog the common bile duct, thereby inhibiting the flow of digestive juices into the intestines and allowing the development of flatulence.

Avoiding Cleansing Reactions

It is widely believed that cleansing reactions are a necessary consequence of purifying the body and cannot long be avoided when any significant amount of cleansing is being done.

The primary message of the author, which carries through in all of my herbal and dietary programs, is that the just-mentioned belief is emphatically not so! In order to control cleansing reactions, all that is needed is a good understanding of the dynamics of the body purification process and the adherence to two simple principles in formulating any dietary or herbal program. Every one of my health programs is distinguished by its ability to deliver results while doing away with all cleansing reactions, except, in some cases, for minor, infrequently occurring, or easily tolerated ones. I am a successful person, and my success has been founded upon my ability to perform in this critical area. No person in the world is, to the best of my knowledge, more of an expert on this subject than I am.

Cleansing reactions may be avoided by adherence to the following two principles. First, keep the rate of cleansing within manageable limits. Second, balance out the aggressive modes of the cleansing agents used with appropriate counteraggressive herbs.

Blood-purifying herbs increase the rate at which toxins are removed from the blood. Lymph-purifying herbs increase the rate in which toxins are removed from the lymph. Provided their amounts are kept at a manageable level, blood-aggressive and lymph-aggressive agents may be used without increasing the toxicity of the blood or lymph by combining them with appropriate quantities of blood-purifying and lymph-purifying herbs. Note, however, that there is a maximum amount of increased blood purification and lymph purification that can be obtained, so that there is a corresponding maximum amount of blood-aggressive and lymph-aggressive activity that can be counterbalanced.

Mucocorrective herbs counteract mucoaggressive responses by flushing softened mucoid out of a confined area. They generally do not possess the powerful mucotriptic activity necessary to dissolve hardened mucoid, but they do complement this type of activity by removing the mucoid once it is softened. The substances removed by mucocorrective herbs are excreted primarily through the liver in the form of bile. Using mucocorrective herbs therefore increases the flow of bile. Because there is a limit to how much bile production can be comfortably tolerated, there are corresponding limits to how much of the mucocorrective herbs should be used and, hence, to how much mucoaggressive activity can be balanced out. Some mucocorrective herbs are blessed thistle, dandelion root, gentian root, and rosemary.

Carminative herbs allay the formation of gas in the intestinal tract. They do so by clearing the common bile duct of the sludge that interferes with the proper flow of digestive juices into the intestines. An appropriate amount of carminative activity should be present in any herbal formula that might otherwise result in flatulence.

At this point, we shall not discuss how to deal with the possibility of deobstruent herbs producing constipated and infrequent bowel movements. This is a matter that will be taken up later when we discuss the actual process of gastrointestinal cleansing in greater detail.

Keeping the rate of cleansing within manageable limits involves the careful selection of which herbs to use. For example, the list of mucotriptic herbs is long, giving one many herbs to choose from. The lists for lymph-purifying and blood-purifying herbs are also long. When devising a combination herbal formula, there are usually many possible combinations to consider.

In some methods of herbal practice, the common procedure is to combine the strongest known herbs having the desired mode of activity. This often results in more aggressive cleansing activity than can be balanced out by counteraggressive herbs. It is no surprise that the person who uses formulas of this kind reaches the conclusion that cleansing reactions are inevitable. In fact, such a belief may lead a person to judge the potency of an herb by its level of aggressive cleansing activity, rather than by a more careful and difficult assessment of its impact upon health. Such an approach will result in a habitual choosing of highly aggressive herbs, even when less aggressive ones might do better at securing the desired results.

In formulating his herbal approach to gastrointestinal cleansing, the author has taken several important steps that result in a highly effective formula having very little tendency to produce cleansing reactions. First, highly aggressive herbs have been avoided. Second, as much as possible, the mucotriptic herbs used are specific to the gastrointestinal tract. This gives a good level of gastrointestinal cleansing activity while minimizing the level of cleansing at other bodily locations. Third, mucosynergistic combinations capable of augmenting the gastrointestinal cleansing activity of the formula have been painstakingly sought. Doing so has been quite fruitful in that the increase in desired activity has been obtained with virtually no increase in mucoaggressive activity. Fourth, the moderate aggressive cleansing activity that would otherwise be present has been balanced out with appropriate counteraggressive herbs.

About Metabolic Activators

In Chapter Three, we mentioned bladderwrack, oatstraw, spirulina plankton, grapes (including raisins and grape juice), irish moss, yeast, and vinegar as being metabolic activators and discussed each. Of these, oatstraw, spirulina plankton, grapes, and irish moss are mucoaggressive. All except spirulina plankton are blood aggressive. And spirulina plankton is highly lymph aggressive.

About Blood-Purifying Agents

The author uses the term "blood purifier" in a more strict sense than will be found in most herbal writings. For the author, a *blood purifier* is an agent that will counterbalance blood-aggressive activity by promoting the removal of waste substances such as uric acid from the blood. Nothing more is meant by the term. Some blood purifiers are balm of gilead buds, birch bark, blue flag root, burdock root, butternut bark, cabbage, chaparral, couchgrass, devil's claw root, echinacea root, garlic, gentian root, iceberg lettuce (use or dehydrate before any milky juice or narcotic properties develop), oregon grape root, rosemary, and yellow dock root. Of these burdock root, garlic, and gentian root are lymph aggressive.

Historically, there have been a number of modes of herbal activity that were believed to be due to purifying the blood. For example, skin eruptions were considered to be caused by excesssive toxins in the blood seeking to escape through the skin. Therefore, an herb that was healing to skin diseases would be labeled a blood purifier. Yes, skin diseases are due to excessive toxins; but these toxins do not necessarily come from the blood. Even to this day, there are writings that do not distinguish the lymph from the blood when speaking of the circulation, and we commonly find symptoms of a toxic lymph being referred to as symptoms of a toxic blood. In line with this practice, we find herbs that are beneficial to the lymph glands being designated as blood purifiers. Finally, there is the idea of alterative herbs; these gradually improve overall health and restore normal bodily functions, supposedly by purifying the blood. To perform such a feat requires the purification of the entire body, and so alteratives would be better described as body purifiers than blood purifiers. Nevertheless, the terms "alterative" and "blood purifier" are often considered to be synonomous. Mucotriptic herbs make good body purifiers, and so we find many of these being referred to as alteratives or as blood purifiers.

Limiting Factor Removed

A limiting factor to the general acceptance of herbs and other forms of natural healing has been their susceptibility to give rise to cleansing reactions. This has led people to turn largely away from many of Nature's remedies in favor of health-care modalities that suppress symptoms without removing their cause.

Health-care professionals offering natural-healing modalities have been largely unable to meet the challenge of practicing their art while keeping their clients clear of cleansing reactions. Often the approach has been to assert it to be a law of Nature that a person using a natural-healing modality must expect to feel worse before feeling better. The idea behind this approach is to prepare people to persevere through cleansing reactions when they do occur. While a few people may respond in the intended way, this approach serves to discourage the majority of people. People need health-care delivery through natural modalities without serious cleansing reactions, and this is what is finally being made available through the work of the author.

Natural-healing health-care professionals highly agree that most diseases begin with a toxic colon, and that the first and most important step towards improved health is to cleanse the colon. With the publication of this book, the way has finally been prepared for those interested in self-help health care to unhesitatingly begin their trek down the road to renewed health. No longer need one feel uncertain about wanting to embark upon a colon-cleansing program. All may now avail themselves of Nature's design for bodily wholeness, which begins with proper colon care.

Chapter Five

Practical Gastrointestinal and Lymphatic Cleansing

COMPONENTS OF AN EFFECTIVE COLON-CLEANSING PROGRAM

There are three functions which a colon-cleansing program must perform in order to successfully remove all stagnant material from the colon. They are: (1) stop or decrease the ongoing production of mucoid in the alimentary tract; (2) loosen the stagnant material; and (3) remove the loosened material. Let us discuss each of these in turn.

Controlling Mucoid

The degree to which the ongoing production of mucoid needs to be controlled depends upon the strength of the substance used to dissolve the old, hardened mucoid glued inside the colon. The moisture moving through the intestines is only capable of holding a limited amount of mucoid in solution. If all of the mucoid-dissolving powers of a colon-cleansing program get used up by the fresh mucoid being created, then there will be nothing left to dissolve the hardened mucoid. In this case, all that will happen is that no new deposits will be laid down. If the ongoing production of mucoid is somewhat less, then there will be a small surplus of mucoid-dissolving activity acting upon the hardened deposits. Colon cleansing will proceed, but at a very slow rate. If the ongoing production of mucoid is stopped, then all of the available mucoid-dissolving activity will be used upon the stagnant mucoid, and colon cleansing will proceed at its maximum possible rate.

Most bona-fide colon-cleansing programs stipulate either fasting or a totally nonmucoidforming diet of vegetables, fruits, and sometimes sprouts be adhered to. This has the effect of stopping the ongoing production of mucoid in the alimentary tract.

The gastrointestinal cleansing program given here uses a combination of lactobacteria supplementation when needed, eating sun chokes or drinking cabbage juice if desired, and lowering the mucoidforming food intake as necessary to control the production of alimentary tract mucoid. This way, the whole burden need not be placed upon dietary restrictions alone. In addition, the importance of the metabolic rate in determining mucoid production has been brought to light, and a simple technique for measuring one's relative metabolic rate has been given. The procedure given here is powerful enough that, in most cases, a fairly highly mucoidforming diet may be eaten and gastrointestinal cleansing will still proceed. Once it has been communicated how increasing the balance of mucoidforming versus countermucoid influences and a low metabolic rate slow down the gastrointestinal cleansing process, final dietary discretion is left to the person seeking benefit from the program.

Loosening Stagnant Material

In Chapter Four, we discussed the usefulness of mucotriptic herbs for loosening stagnant material in the colon. Let us briefly discuss three other agents used for this purpose but not previously mentioned.

Bentonite, pumice, and clay: Bentonite and pumice are special varieties of volcanic ash. Bentonite, pumice, and some varieties of clay are quite effective at loosening stagnant material. Their mode of activity is, however, quite different from that of the author's herbal formula. The herbal formula dissolves hardened mucoid layer by layer. As it redissolves, the mucoid swells up with water to its original bulk and passes out of the body as a soft mass. Bentonite, pumice, and clay, on the other hand, lift hardened mucoid off the colon wall without dissolving, moisturizing, or softening it. Sometimes huge chunks or strips that are hard as a rubber tire are set free, only to serve as a source of obstruction to the through passage of fresh feces. Because the colon was designed to pass soft, moist, easily formed substances and not hard, rubbery ones, a person should proceed slowly and cautiously when using bentonite, pumice, or clay products.

Coffee: The use of coffee enemas for colon cleansing is fairly widespread. Coffee is not nearly as powerful for this purpose, however, as many of the mucotriptic herbs. It must be taken rectally, as taking coffee orally has no colon-cleansing effect.

Water: This is the solvent used in colonic irrigations. Its weak but persistent solvent activity will remove some but not all of the stagnant material from the colon.

Removing Loosened Material

Colon cleansing will proceed much more quickly if we remove old feces as soon as they begin to loosen, rather than wait until they are loose enough to just flow out. As hardened mucoid gets redissolved, it becomes sticky again. The reintroduction of all this sticky mucoid into the flow of material through the colon can, and oftentimes does, produce highly constipated and infrequent bowel movements. To wait for all of this mucoid to dissolve enough that the bowels move regularly again may take a very long time. It is therefore important to remove loosened material quickly.

Psyllium husks (Plantago ovata (Forsk.); Plantaginaceae) are unsurpassed at removing loosened material. They swell enormously with water, forming a bulky, jellylike medium that is amazing for its ability to absorb large quantities of sticky, gluey mucoid and still retain its slippery, nonsticky, lubricating nature. This converts the sticky, constipated redissolved feces into a moist, bulky, and nonsticky mass which can then pass easily from the body. Psyllium husks also aid the activity of the mucotriptic agents by holding considerable extra water in the colon. This water is much needed for softening the dehydrated mucoid.

Water is also a thoroughly reliable agent for removing loosened feces from the colon. A few quick two-quart enemas will remove all the loose material without the long waiting period required for substances taken orally to act on the colon.

SURVEY OF COLON-CLEANSING ALTERNATIVES

Let us take a look at some colon-cleansing schemes available today. Each contains provisions for controlling mucoid, loosening old feces, and removing loosened material.

Olive-oil fast: For several days the person ingests only water plus two tablespoons olive oil with a half cup orange juice taken four to five times per day. If the bowels do not move shortly after the fast is broken, water enemas are used to reestablish bowel regularity. Here fasting is used to stop the ongoing production of mucoid, olive oil is used to loosen stagnant material, and enemas are used if necessary to remove loosened material. This procedure usually gets a quantity of old feces out, but it would have to be repeated many times before the colon became completely clean.

Volcanic-ash fast: Perform a seven-day juice fast during which psyllium husks and either pumice or bentonite (both volcanic products) are taken several times a day. In some versions of this program, clay is used in place of the volcanic ash. In one version, the person on the program must also take a two-quart, hour-long coffee enema each day, during which the colon is massaged while the coffee is being let in in small amounts at a time. These programs use fasting to stop the ongoing production of mucoid, volcanic ash or clay and sometimes also coffee and massage to loosen stagnant material, and psyllium husks and sometimes enemas to remove the loosened material. Several seven-day fasts are needed to remove all old feces.

Colonic irrigations: These are actually just sophisticated enemas using special equipment whereby water can enter the colon and feces can be expelled simultaneously to far exceed what can be accomplished with a home-style enema bag. The person receiving the benefit or a skilled operator should control the equipment. In colonic irrigations, water is used both for loosening and removing the old feces. As far as controlling mucoid is concerned, we must understand that colonic irrigations are usually given by hire and so mucoid control is left to the discretion of the client. However, if we consult Dr. Norman Walker, today's foremost authority on colonic irrigations, we find a strong insistence upon the necessity for a vegetable, fruit, and juice diet in order for colonic irrigations to be of full benefit. Even so, it takes dozens of colonic irrigations performed over more than a year's time to get the maximum benefit from this procedure.

Colonic irrigations are different in scope and impact from the author's colon-cleansing program in two important ways. First, a major part of their effectiveness is due to the enema effect, which was discussed in Chapter Two. Because they evoke the enema effect, colonic irrigations can be of health benefit even after the colon has been completely cleansed. In this way, colonic irrigations offer something that cannot be obtained simply by cleansing the colon alone. While a clean colon prevents the long-term negative reflex activity upon the body caused by a toxic colon, it does not generate the powerful short-term positive reflex impulse upon the body afforded by colonic irrigations. Second, colonic irrigations alone will not remove the most hardened mucoid from the colon. In Chapter Two, we said that the stagnant material in the colon is of two types. There is the putrefactive material that is still moist and decaying. This colonic irrigations will remove. But then there is the hardened postputrefactive material that is very dry and glued into the body. This needs to be loosened by a powerful solvent before it will ever budge. The author has seen people who, after having had numerous colonic irrigations, still passed large amounts of old feces using the program in this book. We are not trying to say that colonic irrigations are a useless technique; they are quite powerful in their own sphere of activity. While there is some overlap between colonic irrigations and the author's gastrointestinal cleansing program, there are important differences also.

Colonic irrigations harmonize well with the author's colon-cleansing program. While the program is sufficient by itself to completely cleanse the colon, faster progress can be made by supplementing it with weekly colonic irrigations. Colonic irrigation therapists have consistently been amazed at the quantity of old feces passed during irrigations performed in conjuction

Be Notified
of Additional Activities
# of Robert Gray

Now you can follow all aspects of Robert Gray's work—simply and easily

Each day Robert Gray receives letters from readers of *The Colon Health Handbook*. These people are enthusiastic about his work and repeatedly ask about the availability of additional ways to benefit by his ability to help people. Many sense Robert Gray's commitment to promote better health through wholistic and natural means and would like to see more people touched by his work. Because he knows that there are thousands more people like these, Robert Gray now offers to send to all who are interested in any aspect of his work:

- *Advance notice when new books being written by Robert Gray are completed*

- *Articles and personal messages from Robert Gray*

- *Notification of public and media appearances by Robert Gray*

- *Information on new self-help programs developed by Robert Gray*

- *Information about seminars and trainings when offered by Robert Gray*

- *Ways those interested can participate in Robert Gray's efforts to bring better health to the world*

Identify yourself as a friend of Robert Gray and his work. Your name and address will be kept confidential and will not be added to any other mailing list. Simply fill out and send in this handy card today.

Please Print Clearly

Name _____

Address _____

_____

_____ Zip _____

Emerald Publishing
P. O. Box 11830
Reno, Nevada 89510

with the author's program.

When one receives a colonic irrigation, there are two precautions of which to be aware. The first precaution is to avoid receiving an irrigation given with chlorinated water. Rather, it is best to locate a facility that uses purified water. As discussed in Chapter Six, irrigations with chlorinated water can destroy the friendly lactobacteria present in the colon. Operators who use chlorinated water often try to compensate for this by encouraging their clients to eat plenty of yogurt or kefir to replace the destroyed lactobacteria. These foods are highly mucoidforming, however, and eating them is essentially counterproductive to good health. When the balance of the intestinal flora has been upset, use the rejuvelac procedure given in Chapter Six rather than eat yogurt or kefir. The second precaution in connection with colonic irrigations is to realize that they are capable of producing cleansing reactions. The enema effect is a natural-healing phenomenon wherein toxins are stirred up all over the body. This does not mean one should avoid colonic irrigations, as it is good to rid one's body of whatever toxins are present. However, moderation should be exercised in order to avoid cleansing reactions of an intensity that is difficult to tolerate. When a single long colonic irrigation is likely to result in too strong of a cleansing reaction, it is better to take two or three shorter irrigations over a period of time. And when three irrigations per week are too intense, it is better to reduce the frequency to one or two per week.

A COMPREHENSIVE GASTROINTESTINAL AND LYMPHATIC CLEANSING PROGRAM

In spite of the many benefits of intestinal cleansing, the author's experience as Director of the Food For Health Institute has clearly indicated that few people will persist at a program similar to any of those just outlined long enough to completely cleanse the colon. It seems that everybody leads a busy life and is only willing to devote a minimum amount of time and effort to any single endeavor. When seeking professional assistance, an individual needs not only a ready source of knowledge, but also streamlined methods for the practical application of that knowledge. These methods should take only small amounts of time and be easy to perform.

Accordingly, the author set out to develop an intestinal cleansing program which would (1) avoid the use of fasting, enemas, or other difficult procedures; (2) require only a few minutes per day; (3) be suitable for use along with diets other than that taught at the Institute; and (4) be performable continuously on a day-by-day basis until the colon was completely cleansed. The result has been the emergence of a program that took seven years to develop. In most cases, it meets all of the specified requirements. It has been highly appreciated by those who have followed it.

There are three simple parts to the program, namely, (1) a tableted intestinal cleansing formula that is taken up to four times per day; (2) an intestinal bulking agent taken two to four times per day; and (3) about four to five minutes of skin brushing performed once per day. Because everything taken into the body with this program enters through the mouth and not through the anus, it cleanses not only the colon but the entire alimentary tract. Let us take a closer look at each of the three parts.

The tableted intestinal cleansing formula contains chickweed, irish moss, cloves, plantain, rosemary, bayberry bark, and corn silk extract. The intestinal bulking agent contains psyllium husks, plantago endosperm, plantago embryo, and cloves. The tableted intestinal cleansing formula and to a lesser extent the intestinal bulking agent act to loosen stagnant material, while the intestinal bulking agent is exceptionally effective at removing the loosened material. Together they make up the author's herbal formula for gastrointestinal cleansing. Let us discuss the various modes of activity in this formula.

Mucotriptic: There are six mucotriptic herbs used in the author's formula which together form a strong mucosynergistic relationship that is capable of dissolving the most hardened stagnant mucoid. Each of these six herbs when used alone, regardless of the quantity, is quite feeble compared to the effectiveness of the combination. Furthermore, the mucoaggressive activity of these herbs is quite low. Two of the six herbs are without mucoaggressive activity, while that of the remaining four is slight and seldom ever felt.

Bowel regulator: *Bowel regulators* exert a counterbalancing tendency upon both constipation and diarrhea. We have already mentioned how dissolving old mucoid back into the flow of material passing through the intestines tends to make the stools more constipated. Let us now also mention that the liver tends to secrete more bile when cleansing herbs are being taken, and that extra bile can give rise to diarrhea. Therefore, both constipated stools and diarrhea can occur during a colon-cleansing program. Four of the herbs in the author's formula act together to provide good bowel regulator activity.

Lymph purifier: There are two lymph-purifying herbs in the formula which together provide an extra measure of lymph-purifying activity beyond what is necessary to counterbalance the single lymph-aggressive herb present.

Blood purifier: A generous amount of blood-purifying activity is provided in the formula to counterbalance the blood-aggressive activity of the two lymph-purifying herbs.

Mucocorrective: A generous amount of mucocorrective activity is provided in the formula to counterbalance the moderate mucoaggressive activity of the mucotriptic herbs.

Carminative: While the herbs in the formula by themselves have little tendency to produce flatulence, a generous amount of carminative herb is present to allay any flatulence arising as a cleansing reaction. This carminative herb is also soothing and settling to the stomach and the entire intestinal tract.

Each ingredient in this formula possesses multiple herbal activities, which, in most cases, interact with the herbal activities of the other ingredients. The delicate balancing of these properties relults in a formula which possesses all of the factors necessary to be highly effective while, at the same time, is gentle and minimizes the tendency for cleansing reactions to arise. It is the combining of the correct ingredients in delicately-balanced ratios that took the author years to determine which accounts for the outstanding nature of this formula.

Skin brushing is the primary lymphatic-cleansing modality. It acts in combination with the intestinal cleansing formula, whose mucotriptic properties have a softening effect upon hardened lymph mucoid.

The items needed to perform the author's intestinal cleansing program are widely available through a variety of sources.

Starting The Gastrointestinal Cleansing

People vary markedly in their sensitivity to this intestinal cleansing program. The amount of intestinal cleansing formula and intestinal bulking agent required for an effective cleansing differs for everyone. Also, as the intestinal cleansing progresses, there is less toxic material present, so that larger and larger doses become appropriate.

The chart on a nearby page shows the progression of recommended dosage levels. Because the intestinal bulking agent has some intestinal cleansing activity even when used without the intestinal cleansing formula tablets, everyone should begin the program with a period of time taking the intestinal bulking agent only. Always start at the Initial Test Level of the chart. Approximately 70 to 80% of the people are able to advance to Level E after three or more days on the Initial Test Level. However, some people need to progress through Levels A through D before going on to Level E in order to have a smooth and comfortable experience of the cleansing process. As the chart indicates, you begin by taking two level teaspoons of the intestinal bulking agent two times per day. If you do not feel comfortable at this level, or if the frequency or quantity of your bowel movements is less, discontinue this level immediately and wait three days. Then resume the program at Level A. If you continue to feel comfortable with the Initial Test dosage for three to four days, move immediately to Level E, using the dosage of the intestinal cleansing formula and intestinal bulking agent indicated.

For every level teaspoon of intestinal bulking agent you take, drink an 8-ounce glass of liquid along with it. The glass should hold 8 ounces when completely filled to the brim, so that you will actually drink about 7 ounces.

The best way to drink the liquid when taking two level teaspoons intestinal bulking agent is to mix all of the intestinal bulking agent in the first glass of liquid and to follow it immediately with a second glass of liquid which is used to take the tableted intestinal cleansing formula. When using the intestinal bulking agent, drink it immediately after stirring it into whatever liquid you are taking it with. Do so because, if the mixture is allowed to sit, it may become too thick to drink. Do not be concerned if the intestinal bulking agent forms into little clumps without dispersing. Once inside the body, they will all eventually absorb large amounts of moisture, provided enough moisture is present.

Always begin at the Initial Test Level and follow all instructions given herein whenever you initiate or reinitiate taking the author's formulas. Start at the Initial Test Level regardless of how good your diet may be. Start at the Initial Test Level even if you have been doing any other form of intestinal cleansing. Start at the Initial Test Level if more than three weeks have elapsed since you last took the author's formulas. If less than three weeks have elapsed, go back one or two dosage levels when resuming the author's formulas.

While performing Level G or beyond of the program, try to always take the formulas four times per day. One way to do this is to use them with each meal and at bedtime. If your schedule does not allow you to space the doses evenly, then as little as three hours between doses is permissible. Taking the formulas only three instead of four times per day requires that you do so for a 33% greater number of days to accomplish the same amount of cleansing.

The formulas may be taken before, after, or inbetween meals. When taken before meals, the intestinal bulking agent tends to decrease the appetite because it swells and so partially fills the empty stomach. This may be helpful to persons desiring to lose weight. If you prefer to avoid this effect, take the formulas after your meal.

Controlling Your Progress On the Program

You should control your progress from level to level by noting the frequency and quantity of your bowel movements. If you are on too low a dosage level, these movements will be similar to what you normally experienced prior to starting the program. As you progress to higher dosage levels, the frequency and quantity of your bowel movements will increase. However, if you go to too high a dosage level prematurely, they will begin to decrease again. Therefore, you should stay at the dosage level which produces the best increase in the frequency and quantity of your bowel movements while allowing you to feel comfortable in other respects.

When you find you are not ready for one dosage level and return to the previous one, stay on the one you returned to long enough to double the amount of time spent on that level so far. For example, if you spent 3 days

Recommended Dosages

Dosage Level	Level Teaspoons Intestinal Bulking Agent Per Dose	Tablets Intestinal Cleansing Formula Per Dose	Number of Doses Per Day	Minimum Days At This Level
Initial Test	2	none	2	3
A	1	none	1	3
B	1	none	2	3
C	2	none	1	3
D	2	½	1	3
E	2	½	2	3
F	2	1	2	10
G	2	1	4	14
H	2	2	4	42
I	2	3	4	n/a

Important: with every dose drink an 8-ounce glass of liquid for each level teaspoon Intestinal Bulking Agent.

on Level E and then return to it after trying Level F, you would then spend another 3 days on Level E. If you then test Level F and return to Level E again, you would then spend 6 more days on Level E before attempting Level F again.

You will find the frequency of your bowel movements varies throughout the program. For some people, the frequency may reach up to four or five movements per day at some point during the program. The length of time needed to stay on each level varies from a few days to several weeks. The maximum rate at which anyone should progress from dosage level to dosage level is as follows: 3 days at the Initial Test Level; 3 days at Level E; 10 days at Level F; 2 weeks at Level G; 6 weeks at Level H; and Level I until completion of the program. Not that these are the minimum amounts of time the fastest-progressing person should stay on each level. Most people wil be slower than the fastest-progressing person, so do not hesitate to spend longer on each level (except Level I) if at all appropriate.

Persons who need to start the program at Level A will find they need to spend 3 to 21 days on each of Levels A through D. When such people progress to Levels E, F, and G, the minimum time on each of these levels should be whichever is greater between the values given in the preceding paragraph for these levels and the average amount of time spent on Levels A through D. For example, if you spend 46 days on Levels A through D, the average is 12 days per level. Your minimums would then be 12 days for Level E, 12 days for Level F, and 2 weeks for Level G.

Possible Cleansing Reactions

Cleansing reactions of any consequence are generally not to be expected while following this program. However, we will here indicate how to control a cleansing reaction when one does arise and mention ones that might occur.

Cleansing reactions arise when the rate of cleansing is higher than the body can easily tolerate. Decreasing the rate of cleansing to within comfortable limits is always a technique for controlling a cleansing reaction. Therefore, if you are experiencing a cleansing reaction on one level of the program, you should decrease to a level where the reaction is no longer a problem. Let us now take a closer look at the process associated with cleansing reactions on this gastrointestinal cleansing program.

The stagnant mucoid within the intestinal tract possesses varying degrees of hardness. It does not take large amounts of mucotriptic activity to begin dissolving the relatively soft putrefactive mucoid present at the beginning of a colon-cleansing program. However, a good measure of mucotriptic activity will eventually be necessary to finally remove the most hardened postputrefactive deposits. Because this program possesses mucotriptic activity sufficient to remove the most hardened postputrefactive deposits, using larger doses in the beginning can easily result in an uncomfortably high rate of cleansing. Furthermore, as the cleansing progresses, the colon becomes steadily more efficient at detoxifying the lymph, thereby making it easier for toxins throughout the body to escape without producing adverse reactions. Accordingly, the tendency for a cleansing reaction to be present is strongest towards the beginning of this program and decreases steadily as the cleansing is completed. Therefore, to control a cleansing reaction, use the smaller dosage levels at the beginning and proceed stepwise to the larger dosage levels with the passage of time. The length of time necessary to remain on any level should be dictated by the comfort of the person performing the program, but in no case should exceed the minimums given in the previous subsection of this chapter.

One cleansing reaction possible on this program is constipated and infrequent bowel movements. These occur because more mucoid is being dissolved into the flow of material passing through the intestines than can be absorbed by the intestinal bulking agent. They are a sign either that too highly mucoidforming of a diet is being eaten, or that stagnant mucoid is being dissolved too quickly. They are more likely to occur when there is a low metabolic rate. They can arise as a result of drinking less than the recommended amount of liquid with the intestinal bulking agent. They can also occur as a result of the intestinal cleansing formula being used either without the intestinal bulking agent or with too little of it. When such is the case, the stagnant mucoid will be softened faster than the intestinal bulking agent is removing it. This may not seem to cause a problem in the beginning, but will eventually create a situation where the intestines contain large amounts of softened but still stagnant mucoid. The point will finally be reached where the intestinal bulking agent is drawing more softened mucoid into the flow of material passing through the intestines than it can absorb, resulting in constipated bowel movements.

Whenever there is a tendency towards constipated and infrequent bowel movements while following this program, immediately return to the Initial Test dosage level until regularity has been reestablished. Be sure you are drinking the recommended amount of liquid with each dose of intestinal bulking agent. Consider the possibility that what you have been using as a level teaspoon of intestinal bulking agent is actually less. Purchase a measuring spoon marked "1 teaspoon" and use that henceforth to measure the intestinal bulking agent. When the consitipation passes, advance from the Initial Test Level to Level E, and then proceed stepwise to the largest dosage level you previously attained without a constipation problem, remaining on each level for 2 to 3 days. Also note that if a quick resolution to a bout of constipation is desired, the enema procedure given in the next chapter or a colonic irrigation may be used. To prevent the problem from reoccuring, follow the recommended dosages in stepwise sequence and do not exceed the maximum rates given earlier for progressing from dosage level to dosage level. To speed progress to the full Level H dosages, prepare and use some rejuvelac as detailed in Chapter Six of this book. Doing so supplies a large amount of friendly lactobacteria whose digestive enzymes and lactic acid are very effective at breaking down excess mucoid, thereby lessening the tendency toward constipated bowel movements. Eating sun chokes or drinking cabbage juice daily, as discussed in Chapter Three, in combination with taking rejuvelac daily can further lessen this tendency.

Women sometimes experience a shortening or lengthening of a menstrual cycle while on this program. This normally poses no difficulty as long as one understands that the pattern of ovulation may also change, invalidating any birth control technique involving knowing or estimating one's fertility period.

Occasionally there is a feeling of unsettledness in the stomach shortly after the intestinal bulking agent is taken. It is usually worse after the first dose in the morning or the last dose in the evening has been taken on an empty stomach. The intestinal bulking agent itself does not disturb the system. The unsettledness is due to large amounts of softened toxic material being moisturized by the intestinal bulking agent and reintroduced into the flow of material through the alimentary tract. It is usually the result of a pattern of having taken the intestinal cleansing formula tablets without a sufficient amount of intestinal bulking agent. Doing so allows an excess accumulation of loosened toxins which are rapidly redissolved when the intestinal bulking agent is taken. Follow the procedure for constipation given earlier if this problem arises. Whenever any difficulty is likely, avoid taking the intestinal bulking agent and the intestinal cleansing formula on an empty stomach. If there is a particular time of day during which the difficulty occurs, omit any doses of intestinal bulking agent and intestinal cleansing formula scheduled to be taken during that time. When this problem does occur, it will not persist indefinitely, but it will disappear once the toxins that are dissolving so quickly are cleared away.

Skin brushing acts more to control cleansing reactions than to produce them. This is so because of its lymph-purifying effect. When one desires to bring a cleansing reaction under control, it is better to increase the skin brushing rather than decrease it.

More On Determining Optimal Dosage Levels

The most desirable or *optimal dosage level* is one that allows intestinal cleansing to proceed at the fastest possible rate while the individual still remains clear of substantial cleansing reactions. Such a dosage level will usually correspond to the minimum dosage level required to assure the passage of at least some old feces with nearly every bowel movement. Going significantly beyond this level will usually slow down the emptying out of old fecal matter by producing constipated and infrequent bowel movements.

When the body weight differs 40 to 50% or more from 125 pounds, dosages should be adjusted so as to be approximately proportional to body weight. For example, a 45- to 75-pound child would take 1 level teaspoon intestinal bulking agent for every 2 teaspoons listed in the chart and ½ tablet intestinal cleansing formula for every 1 tablet listed in the chart. Similarly, a 180- to 220-pound person with a large frame would take 3 level teaspoons intestinal bulking agent for every 2 teaspoons listed in the chart and 1½ tablets intestinal cleansing formual for every 1 tablet listed in the chart. When making these adjustments, be careful never to allow the proportion of intestinal bulking agent to intestinal cleansing formula to be less than stated in the chart. Overweight persons should use dosages appropriate to their ideal weight. This is so because excess fat does not increase the size of the gastrointestinal tract.

Who Should Not Attempt The Program

There are no counterindications specific to children past the age of weaning performing this intestinal cleansing program. However, with children as with adults, care should always be taken to keep the dosages below the point where substantial cleansing reactions result.

Pregnant women are advised against performing this gastrointestinal cleansing program unless with the recommendation and close supervision of a competent physician.

Persons with any form of Inflammatory Bowel Disease, such as Crohn's Disease, Regional Ileitis, or Ulcerative Colitis should not attempt this program. All of these conditions are subject to cleansing reactions in the form of intensification of a preexisting symptom. Because of the severity of symptoms in these cases, such people would be better advised to work on improving their diet when approaching natural health care practices. Skin brushing and the intestinal bulking agent may prove tolerable, but the intestinal cleansing formula tablets should not be taken by these people.

Pomegranates and pomegranate juice can be extremely irritating to the colon. The author recommends they never be eaten at any time, whether on or off any his intestinal cleansing program.

Expected Responses

The stagnant matter in the colon is of two types. First, there is the stagnant putrefactive matter. When expelled, it emits a characteristic old feces odor that is much stronger than that of the typical daily bowel movement. Second, there is the postputrefactive matter. This is very hardened and is beyond the state of putrefying any further. It has little odor and is usually grey, black, dark brown, or dark green in color. Most of the putrefactive matter is usually expelled within the first few weeks of following the program. It is easy to recognize by its characteristic odor. The postputrefactive matter usually takes longer to eliminate completely.

While following the program, you should have two or more bowel movements per day. Assuming you are performing skin brushing as outlined below, you will pass jellylike lymph mucoid varying in color from nearly clear through white or yellow to dark brown. During the first few weeks of the program, the elimination of old putrefactive matter will be discernable by its characteristic odor. Much of the old feces being eliminated will have the form of irregularly shaped mucoid ropes and knots. By the fourth or fifth week of the program, you will begin to pass postputrefactive matter. You will pass grey postputrefactive mucoid, as well as many shades of brown postputrefactive feces. Much of the postputrefactive matter being eliminated will be noticeable by the presence of two or more shades of feces in the same bowel movement. Some of the postputrefactive matter will be nearly black in color. It may come out in huge chunks or in little pieces.

Around the fourth week or so of the program, whatever parasites are present will be expelled. They imbed themselves in the putrefactive matter, which typically takes 3 to 5 weeks to eliminate. Once the putrefactive matter has been eliminated, the parasites have nothing left to hang onto and will be expelled. These vary from tiny threadworms to large, flat tapeworms over a foot long. The most common are the tan-colored roundworms.

Persons who have followed a very pure nonmucoidforming diet for several years will pass little putrefactive matter, but they will find the colon still contains residues of postputrefactive matter. This is because such a diet stops the depositing of new putrefactive matter, allowing any putrefactive matter present to finally become postputrefactive. Diet alone will not, however, remove the postputrefactive matter that began accumulating shortly after birth.

When you begin taking the intestinal bulking agent, your abdomen will swell considerably. This happens because the old feces are swelling up with water in the process of being softened. Weight loss may seem slow compared to the amount of old feces eliminated because each pound of hardened feces will weigh several pounds when it finally leaves the body. Once all the old feces are removed, your abdomen will not swell even when the intestinal bulking agent is taken. When the gastrointestinal cleansing has been completed and the program stopped, your abdomen will be flatter than ever, and you will feel lighter.

Judging Your Progress

As long as the feces have the characteristic odor of old putrefactive matter, contain an intermingling of different shades and textures, are atypically dark in color, or have shapes other than smooth and cylindrical, old feces are being eliminated. If you are having trouble distinguishing the old feces from the fresh, then take two of the four doses per day of intestinal cleansing formula or intestinal bulking agent with a glass of carrot juice for a few days while keeping away from spinach and other green leafy vegetables high in oxalic acid. This will usually turn the fresh feces a bright orangish brown, making them easy to distinguish from the darker old feces. If no portion of the feces become a bright orangish brown as a result of drinking the carrot juice, this indicates that old feces are still present and are dissolving thoroughly enough to become homogenously mixed with the fresh feces.

When you find bowel movements occurring that contain no noticeable old feces, this usually indicates you should progress to the next greater dosage level providing you will not exceed the maximum rate of progress given earlier in this chapter and provided you feel comfortable doing so.

Once you intestines have been full cleansed, you should notice no more dark colors nor intermingling of shades in your bowel movements, their shape should be smooth and cylindrical, and their frequency will decline towards what was normal when you started the program. Also, you will probably have progressed to Level H or I.

The time required to completely cleanse the colon is typically three months, but this varies much from person to person. A low metabolic rate, a highly mucoidforming diet, increasing age, an extremely mucoidforming dietary history, a debilitated or hereditarily weak colon, longer times spent at the lesser dosage levels, and poor adherence to the program are all factors tending to lengthen the time required. There is an autopsy on record wherein the colon was removed and was found to weigh forty pounds. It will take far longer than the typical three months to cleanse such a colon.

Concluding The Program

Once the colon has been cleansed, it will be possible to maintain a high concentration of lactobacteria there. As discussed in Chapter Two, the friendly bacteria are important for building the blood and are helpful for counteracting flatulence and improving digestion. They are also important for producing bulky, well-lubricated stools. A toxic intestinal tract cannot maintain a high concentration of lactobacteria. Furthermore, in sweeping the intestinal tract clear of lose material, the intestinal bulking agent also removes lactobacteria. For these reasons, one should reimplant the lactobacteria in one's system at the end of the program. When concluding the program, stop the intestinal cleansing formula tablets first, and then gradually eliminate the intestinal bulking agent over a one to two week transition period. During this transition period and for eight to twelve weeks thereafter, take rejuvelac as detailed in Chapter Six. And whenever the feces lack the slipperiness and bulkiness obtained while taking rejuvelac, use rejuvelac to reimplant the lactobacteria in one's system.

Skin Brushing

As discussed in Chapter Two, skin brushing is a highly effective technique for cleansing the lymphatic system. Because the gastrointestinal cleansing softens hardened mucoid in the lymphatic system as well as in the intestines, performing skin brushing concurrently with the gastrointestinal cleansing program improves the skin brushing's effectiveness.

The brush used should be a long-handled, bath-type brush. It is essential that it contain natural vegetable bristles. Synthetic bristles should be strictly avoided. The brush should be kept dry and not used for bathing.

When one performs skin brushing, the body should be dry, and the brush should pass once over every part of the body surface except the face. There should be no back and forth motion, circular motion, scrubbing, nor massaging—one clean sweep does it. The direction of the brushing should generally be towards the lower abdomen. Brush down the neck and trunk and brush up the arms, legs, and buttocks. It is permissible to brush across the top of the shoulders and upper back, as the best contact with the skin is made that way.

Skin brushing should be performed once or, if desired, twice per day. A complete skin brushing takes no longer than four or five minutes and is highly stimulating and invigorating. It would take twenty to thirty minutes of lufa or turkish towel massage to get a similar effect.

It is not uncommon for one's stools to contain large amounts of lymph mucoid a day or two after beginning skin brushing. This just represents an emptying out of the backlog of fresh lymph mucoid present in the lymphatic system and is a lymph-purifying effect. As discussed in Chapter Three, lymphatic cleansing goes much deeper than lymph purifying and will take much more time.

Homeostasis

Homeostasis is the tendency of the body to maintain an equilibrium condition wherein all bodily functions are stabilized at normal levels. The body will gradually neutralize the effect of almost any substance that is repeatedly put into it over a long enough period of time. Most herbs lose all effectiveness when taken over a period of eight to nine months. This may happen because the body develops special enzymes to digest or break down the active principles present in the herb. At other times, the body may develop antibodies in the blood that will neutralize an active principle. When an herb subject to homeostasis (and almost all are) is taken regularly, sensitivity to it decreases linearly until all the herb's effectiveness has been lost. Once full homeostatic resistance has been reached, it takes five to seven years of abstinence from the substance in question before maximum sensitivity is regained. In order to prevent homeostatic resistance from reaching the point where an herb is no longer useful, one should not take the herb more than one third of the time.

In order for this gastrointestinal cleansing program to stay effective for periodic use throughout one's life, one should not perform it more than necessary to keep the alimentary tract cleansed. An initial period of three months is usually sufficient to thoroughly cleanse the colon. Do not, however, extend the initial period beyond five months, after which six months of abstinence should follow. Thereafter, the maximum usage of the program should not exceed two months of gastrointestinal cleansing followed by four months of abstinence. Once the colon is completely cleansed, reperform the program every six to twelve months for the minimum time needed to remove the recent accumulations. Conclude each reperformance of the program with a course of rejuvelac, as discussed under "Concluding The Program" in this chapter.

Skin brushing is also subject to homeostatic resistance. The initial skin brushing should begin with the initial gastrointestinal cleansing and should be performed daily for a period of three months, regardless of how long the gastrointestinal cleansing is performed. Thereafter, skin brushing should be performed twice weekly with three to four days between each brushing. It is best to always perform skin brushing on the same two days of every week.

DIETARY CONSIDERATIONS

The process of gastrointestinal cleansing is often inspiring in the direction of dietary change. As all of the ropey, knotted mucoid empties out of the body day after day, one becomes amazed that so much could possibly have been inside. The person may have heard of mucoidforming foods before, but could never find much evidence of large amounts of mucoid in his or her own body. Seeing is believing, and now for the first time the person sees that what he or she has been hearing about mucoidforming foods is true. Many people who eat a mucoidforming diet will state that their diet does not give them any mucoid. Such people should really be saying that all the mucoid created by their diet never seems to get out of the body.

Mucoidforming foods create mucoid not only in the alimentary tract and lymphatic system, but throughout the entire body as well. Mucoid accumulates in every cell and inbetween all the cells. Therefore, your whole body is permeated with mucoid. Cleansing the stomach, intestines, and lymphatics represents a giant and important step towards good health. However, the body cannot be totally healthy until all excess accumulations of mucoid are cast off. To do so requires the regular adherence to a low-mucoidforming diet.

This gastrointestinal cleansing program provides an ideal opportunity for one to change one's diet. By improving nutrient absorption, it enables one to be satisfied with much lighter foods and less quantity of food than before.

Moreover, when the intestinal bulking agent is used and the old, dry feces start to swell up with moisture, a feeling of fullness is created that further reduces the appetite. When these effects are experienced, the best thing to do is to start omitting the more mucoidforming foods from one's diet while retaining and increasing the less mucoidforming ones.

When done properly, dietary change is a smooth and comfortable experience. As you begin changing your diet, reread the sections in Chapter Three entitled "About Dietary Change" and "Mucoidforming Foods."

There is one very important pitfall that you should avoid when changing your diet. This pitfall is cleansing reactions. Cleansing reactions occur when toxic substances are being expelled from the body tissues faster than the organs of elimination can remove them from the body. When this happens, an excess of toxicity builds up in the blood and lymph. In order to eliminate these excess toxins, the body uses a crisis mechanism to supplement the normal activity of the organs of elimination. Such an occurence is referred to as a healing crisis or cleansing reaction.

Fruits, vegetables, and honey are aggressive cleansing foods. They stir up toxins present in the body tissues, forcing these toxins into the blood and lymph. This is good because we want to rid the body of these toxins. However, it is not good if it happens so fast that cleansing reactions develop.

Because vegetables and fruits are nonmucoidforming foods, eating plenty of them is desirable. Because fruits and honey are generally much more aggressive cleansers than vegetables, it is best to start out eating much more vegetables than fruit. (Note well that cucumbers, squashes, etc. are fruit— see Chapter Three.) Some very highly aggressive vegetables are green onions, leeks, chives, and turnips. Also in the category of extremely aggressive foods are spaghetti squash, fenugreek seeds, fenugreek sprouts, and curry powder. All of these highly aggressive foods are highly susceptible to create cleansing reactions and should be eaten very sparingly. Some relatively nonaggressive fruits are avocadoes and tomatoes; these may be eaten freely like most vegetables.

Mature unsprouted seeds, including pulses, grains, and oily seeds, are cleansing inhibitors. They counteract the aggressive cleansing quality of fruits and vegetables. Sprouted seeds are neutral in cleansing quality. They are neither cleansers nor cleansing inhibitors. Of the mature seeds, grains are easier to digest than either oily seeds or pulses.

The best way to begin eliminating mucoidforming foods from one's diet is to move towards a *toxicless diet* of vegetables, fruits, sprouts, honey if desired, millet once per day, and kelp as a supplement. Dairy products eaten should be only from goats' milk, which is far less mucoidforming than cows' milk. Millet is a grain which is gluten free and far less mucoidforming than wheat, rice, oats, rye, or barley. Such a diet eliminates most mucoidforming foods while the millet controls the aggressive cleansing activity of the fruits, honey, and vegetables. Much health benefit can be attained by following such a diet. To go beyond such a diet too soon by eliminating all mature seeds too rapidly is likely to result in cleansing reactions.

Millet is best prepared by cracking it before cooking it. Add 1 cup of millet plus ¾ cup water to a blender. Start the blender at low speed, then advance to high speed and blend 20 seconds. Select a pan with a well-fitting lid. Pour the contents of the blender into the pan. Rinse the blender clean and pour this into the pan also. Cover the millet with 3 to 4 inches of warm water, and stir several times with one hand. Pause a few seconds to allow the millet to settle, and then pour the water off. Cover the millet again with 3 to 4 inches of warm water, and repeat the rinsing procedure for a total of 6 to 7 times. Without this many rinsings, the millet will be sticky and pasty when it cooks. After the last rinse, be sure the millet has been completely drained of water. Now add 1¼ cups distilled or purified water plus ¾ teaspoon salt if desired, and bring to a boil over high heat. Stir the millet frequently while it is coming to a boil; without doing so some of the millet will stick to the bottom of the pan while the rest of it will be mushy and pasty. Once the millet boils, reduce the heat to a very low level, and simmer for 15 minutes with the lid in place. Serve while hot. Makes 2 to 3 servings. May be eaten with breakfast, lunch, or dinner. When eaten for breakfast, pour a fruit smoothie over the top if desired.

Once the gastrointestinal cleansing program has been completed, a good policy to follow is to try to keep the overall balance of mucoidforming versus countermucoid influences low enough that one usually has at least two bowel movements per day. For most people, this will be attainable by: (1) using the diet recommended in the preceding two paragraphs; (2) using rejuvelac as necessary to build up and maintain a high concentration of lactobacteria within the intestinal tract; and (3) supplementing the above, as detailed in Chapter Three, with added cabbage, cabbage juice, and/or sun chokes if necessary.

Chapter Six

Related Natural-Healing Procedures

LACTOBACTERIA FERMENTS

In Chapter Two, we discussed the intestinal bacteria. We saw that the intestines contained putrefactive bacteria as well as the friendly lactobacteria that help to control the activity of the putrefactive bacteria. We also saw that a number of fermented foods contain substantial quantities of live lactobacteria when freshly fermented, but that after a short period of time only high concentrations of lactic acid and little live lactobacteria are left. Because lactic acid is a waste product of metabolism, it should not be consumed in large quantities. Hence fermented food, when eaten, should be freshly prepared at home and consumed within a day's time.

There are special times when it is important to consume fermented food. One time is after taking antibiotics because these kill all the intestinal tract bacteria. When the antibiotics are stopped, the putrefactive bacteria will quickly reestablish themselves in the alimentary tract because they are present everywhere in the environment. The lactobacteria, however, will often not reestablish themselves for some time unless specific action is taken to reintroduce them into the system. Another case in which essentially all the lactobacteria in the colon can be destroyed is when a colonic irrigation or enema using chlorinated water is received. Chlorine is usually added to municipal tap water in order to keep it free of live bacteria. If one is going to receive a colonic irrigation or enema, it is best to be sure purified water is used, from which any chlorine present has been removed. Otherwise, it may become necessary to reimplant the lactobacteria in one's system. A series of several colonic irrigations using purified water can also remove most of the lactobacteria. In fact, any effective colon-cleansing method will remove lactobacteria in the process of pulling stagnant material out of the colon. As discussed in Chapter Five, one should build up the implantation of lactobacteria in the intestines after performing the author's gastrointestinal cleansing program. Rejuvelac may also be used during the program to augment it or to control constipation. Finally, it is sometimes desirable to aid an extremely debilitated digestion with live lactobacteria, as doing so can sometimes make the difference between death and recovery. This should be done at the beginning of an appropriate natural-healing program involving a proper cleansing and rebuilding diet. It should not be relied upon for habitual symptomatic relief whenever a weak digestion is present.

When lactobacteria are to be taken, the recommended form is that of *cabbage rejuvelac*, which is obtained by fermenting fresh cabbage. We have already noted that the so-called lactobacteria present in milk come from the vegetable matter eaten by cows. Cabbage is a vegetable that is teeming with lactobacteria. No starter is needed for making rejuvelac. Just start one morning by blending together 1¾ cups (420 ml) distilled or purified water plus 3 cups (720 ml) coarsely chopped, loosely packed fresh cabbage. Start the blender at low speed and then advance the blender to high speed and blend for 30 more seconds. Pour into a jar, cover, and let stand at room temperature for 3 days. At this time, strain off the liquid rejuvelac. The initial batch of cabbage rejuvelac takes 3 days to mature, but succeeding batches take 24 hours each. Each morning after straining off the fresh rejuvelac, blend together for 30 seconds at high speed 1½ cups (360 ml) distilled or purified water plus 3 cups (720 ml) coarsely chopped, loosely packed fresh cabbage. Pour into a jar, add ¼ cup (60 ml) of the fresh rejuvelac just strained off, cover, shake, and let stand at room temperature until the next morning. You can also make cabbage rejuvelac without a blender by chopping the cabbage very fine and using 2½ cups (600 ml) finely chopped, closely packed fresh cabbage for every 3 cups (720 ml) coarsely chopped, loosely packed cabbage listed above. The amount of distilled or purified water used should remain unchanged. Persons suffering with Candida may need to start each day's rejuvelac by making a batch to which none of the previous day's rejuvelac is added and which is allowed 3 days to mature. Doing so will minimize the possibility of small amounts of airborne yeast contaminating the rejuvelac, as persons suffering with Candida are extremely yeast intolerant.

Good quality rejuvelac tastes similar to a cross between carbonated water and the whey obtained when making yogurt. Bad quality rejuvelac has a much more putrid odor and taste and should not be consumed. Always avoid using tap water when making rejuvelac because chlorine has been added to it for the purpose of killing bacteria of any kind.

In order to obtain good quality rejuvelac, some environments require the use of a negative-ion generator in the room where the rejuvelac is being made. Doing so has a powerful inhibiting effect upon harmful bacteria, but still allows lactobacteria to multiply freely. The method of activity of this inhibiting effect is due at least in part to removing harmful bacteria from the air. In some environments, it is impossible to obtain good quality rejuvelac otherwise.

Drink each day's rejuvelac during the course of the day by taking ½ cup (120 ml) three times per day, preferably with meals. When taking rejuvelac in conjunction with Level G or beyond of the author's gastrointestinal cleansing program, take ⅜ cup or 3 ounces (90 ml) four times per day with each dose of intestinal cleansing formula and intestinal bulking agent. The rejuvelac may be counted as part of the total quantity of liquid taken with each dose of intestinal cleansing formula and intestinal bulking agent. Refrigerate your rejuvelac if it is to be kept overnight. Discard rather than drink any rejuvelac on hand 24 hours after it is poured off from the wheat berries or cabbage.

To implant a healthy population of lactobacteria in the intestinal tract, 1 to 3 months of taking rejuvelac are required. Keep taking rejuvelac daily for a minimum of one month but for however long necessary until you obtain reasonably bulky, well-lubricated stools on a day-after-day basis while eating a diet moderate in mucoidforming activity. If the stools become much less bulky or less lubricated when the rejuvelac is stopped and no change in diet has been made, the implantation was probably unsuccessful and should be tried again. Including cabbage, cabbage juice, or sun chokes in the diet, as detailed in Chapter Three, while rejuvelac is being taken can greatly assist the lactobacteria implantation process. When rejuvenating the digestion through an appropriate natural-healing program, 2 to 3 months of taking rejuvelac should be performed.

The value of rejuvelac should not be confused with that of freeze-dried acidophilus tablets. Rejuvelac contains live lactobacteria. Once freeze dried, lactobacteria die in a few weeks' time. The count of live lactobacteria may be satisfactory when the freeze-dried acidophilus tablets leave the manufacturer, but very often has fallen to an insignificant level by the time the product reaches the consumer. Furthermore, store-bought liquid acidophilus culture is usually an even less reliable source of live lactobacteria than freeze-dried acidophilus tablets.

COLON REBUILDING

In many cases, colon functioning will be satisfactory once the colon is cleansed, a healthy population of lactobacteria has been implanted, and one adopts a *toxicless diet* of vegetables, fruits, sprouts, honey if desired, millet once per day, and kelp as a supplement. However, when the colon is highly debilitated, colon cleansing will prove to be only a first though essential step when using natural methods to help the body regain the full health of its colon; regular adherence to the toxicless diet mentioned together with the maintenance of a healthy population of lactobacteria in the intestinal tract for a considerable period of time will be necessary for the colon to regain is proper shape and tone.

Reeducation of the defecation responses is of utmost importance to good colon health. When the body is functioning properly, it manifests a *gastrocolic reflex* which prompts the bowels to move each time the stomach is filled. Few people, however, have a bowel movement after every meal, partly because, through toilet training, the gastrocolic reflex has been suppressed. We have been taught at a very early age that it is good to restrain the bowels from moving as much as possible. We wait until the call of Nature is overwhelming before consenting to visit the toilet. To rebuild the defecation responses, you must reverse this behavior. Stop to notice if there is any urge towards a bowel movement after every meal. It is essential that you visit the toilet whenever the slightest inkling of the possibility of a bowel movement arises, even when the sensation felt seems much too feeble for an actual bowel movement to occur. Stay there and wait and excercise the muscles of your abdomen and attempt to have even the smallest quantity of feces expelled. Squatting rather than sitting on the toilet helps bowel movements to come easier. Do so by placing the bare feet on the rim of the toilet rather than on the floor and then lower the buttocks as far as possible in this position. Keep persisting at these practices, together with the adherence to the toxicless diet and the maintenance of a healthy population of lactobacteria in the intestinal tract, and you will slowly but surely reach the point where your bowels move with little effort two to four times per day.

DEALING WITH ACUTE SICKNESSES

In Chapter Two, we discussed acute sicknesses; there we saw that both a toxic lymph and a toxic colon interfere with the body's ability to throw off these conditions. Our aim here is not to give specific treatments for specific diseases, but to show techniques that aid the body's recuperative abilities for overcoming whatever ails it.

During an acute sickness, skin brushing and a set of enemas should be performed one or two times per day. Perform the skin brushing immediately before each set of enemas, making up to four passes over each body surface. The person who is not accustomed to skin brushing regularly should only make one pass over each body surface. This creates a pressure for the lymph mucoid to pass into the colon. As soon as an enema is taken, the channels for the flow open up, allowing a measure of lymphatic detoxification to take place.

When taking an enema, put as much as comfortable of two quarts of water into the body at a time. It is best to use distilled, purified, or spring water when available because the chlorine present in tap water kills the friendly lactobacteria in the colon. Boiling tap water for 30 minutes in an uncovered cooking vessel will also remove chlorine from it. Have the water near body temperature because, if it is too hot or too cold, the impetus to expel it will come quicker. When draining the water into the body, do not elevate the enema syringe too high because doing so will force the water into the body so quickly that an immediate impulse to expel it will result. If you lie flat on the floor, hanging the enema syringe from the height of a door knob will be about right. Once all of the water has entered the body, retain it until the body is ready to expel it. Each set should consist of at least three enemas taken in immediate succession. Even if no feces are passed by taking the enemas, there is still a very powerful reflex response throughout the entire body that gets activated.

During the bedridden parts of an acute sickness, the diet should be limited to totally nonmucoidforming foods. Eating is not important at these times, and no food should be forced for which one has no appetite. Once the bedridden stage is passed, millet may be added to the vegetables, fruits, and sprouts already being eaten.